PLANTS

ISBN: 978-81-7436-751-8

Published in India by
Roli Books in arrangement with
Roli & Janssen BV, The Netherlands
M-75, Greater Kailash-II Market,
New Delhi 110 048, India.
Phone: ++91-11-4068 2000
Fax: ++91-11-29217185
Email: info@rolibooks.com
Website: www.rolibooks.com

Editor: Richa Burman
Design: Supriya Saran
Pre-press: Naresh Mondal, Jyoti Dey
Production: Naresh Nigam

Printed and bound in China

PLANTS

WHY YOU CAN'T LIVE WITHOUT THEM

B.C. WOLVERTON

KOZABURO TAKENAKA

Lustre Press
Roli Books

This book is dedicated to our wives, Yvonne and Katsuko, for they are partners in our careers as well as in life. Their working alongside us has made our careers more enjoyable. It is Katsuko's design creativity that has helped bring 'Ecology Gardens' to the forefront. We are especially grateful to Yvonne, without whom this book would not have been possible, for it is her countless hours spent before the computer screen that finally produced our manuscript. It was also her goal to leave a written legacy for Justin and Emily of their grandfather's achievements toward helping to make our environment a better place for them and others to live in.

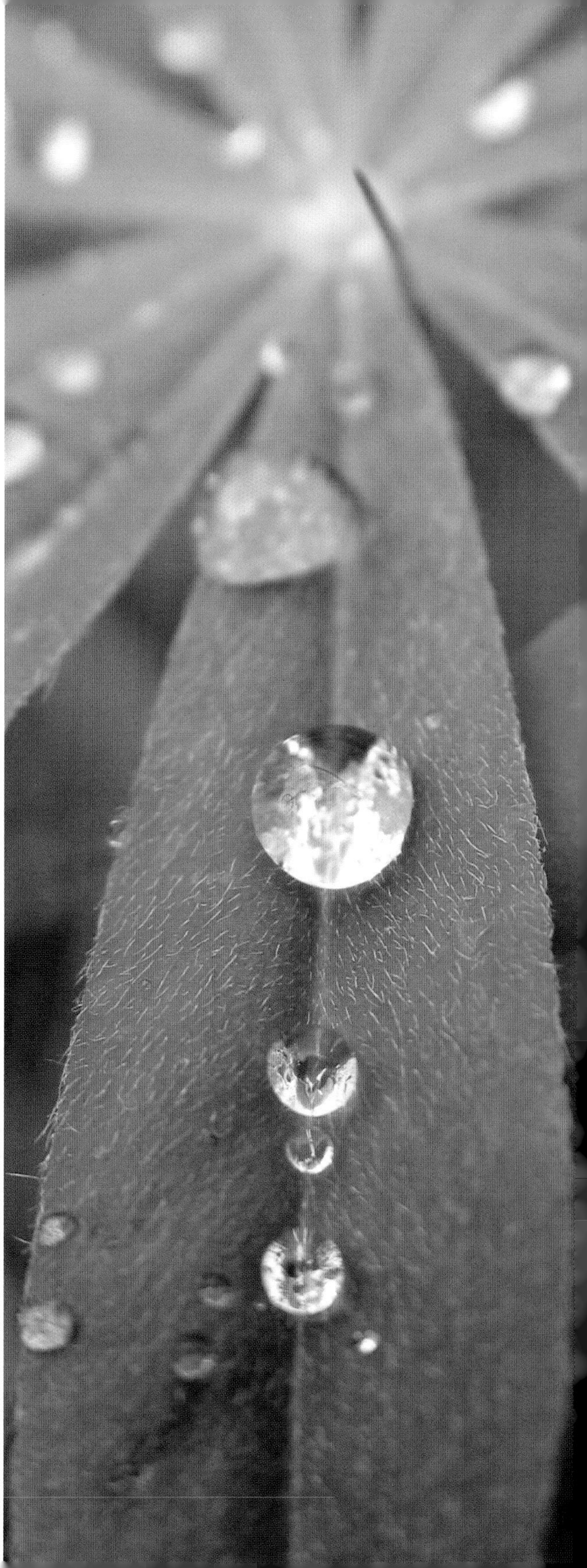

Acknowledgements

We would like to gratefully acknowledge the contributions made by the following: John Wolverton for his many research contributions; the staff at Takenaka Garden Afforestation, Inc.; Tomoo Ryushi, Ph.D, Tokyo Metropolitan University; National Aeronautics and Space Administration at the John C Stennis Space Center, MS; Actree Corporation, Mattoh City, Japan; David Liu, Foliage Design Systems, Orlando, FL; Shane Pliska, Planterra Corporation, West Bloomfield, MI; Beatriz Garces, First Foliage LLC, Homestead, FL; Gaylord Opryland Resort, Nashville, TN; Stuart Rose, Ph.D, Poquoson, VA; Green Plants for Green Buildings (formerly Plants at Work), Ukiah, CA; Professor Kazuo Yamasaki, Teikyo Heisei University, Uruido, Japan; City of Chicago, IL; Andre Trawick, Henderson, KY; Mason Edmunds, Edmunds International; and Kamal Meattle, CEO, Paharpur Business Centre and Software Technology Incubator Park, New Delhi, India.

Our thanks go to our editor, Richa Burman for it was her attention to detail and accuracy that led us to put forth our best efforts. We would also like to extend a special thanks to Priya Kapoor for guiding us through the publishing process. We are grateful to both for their patience and assistance.

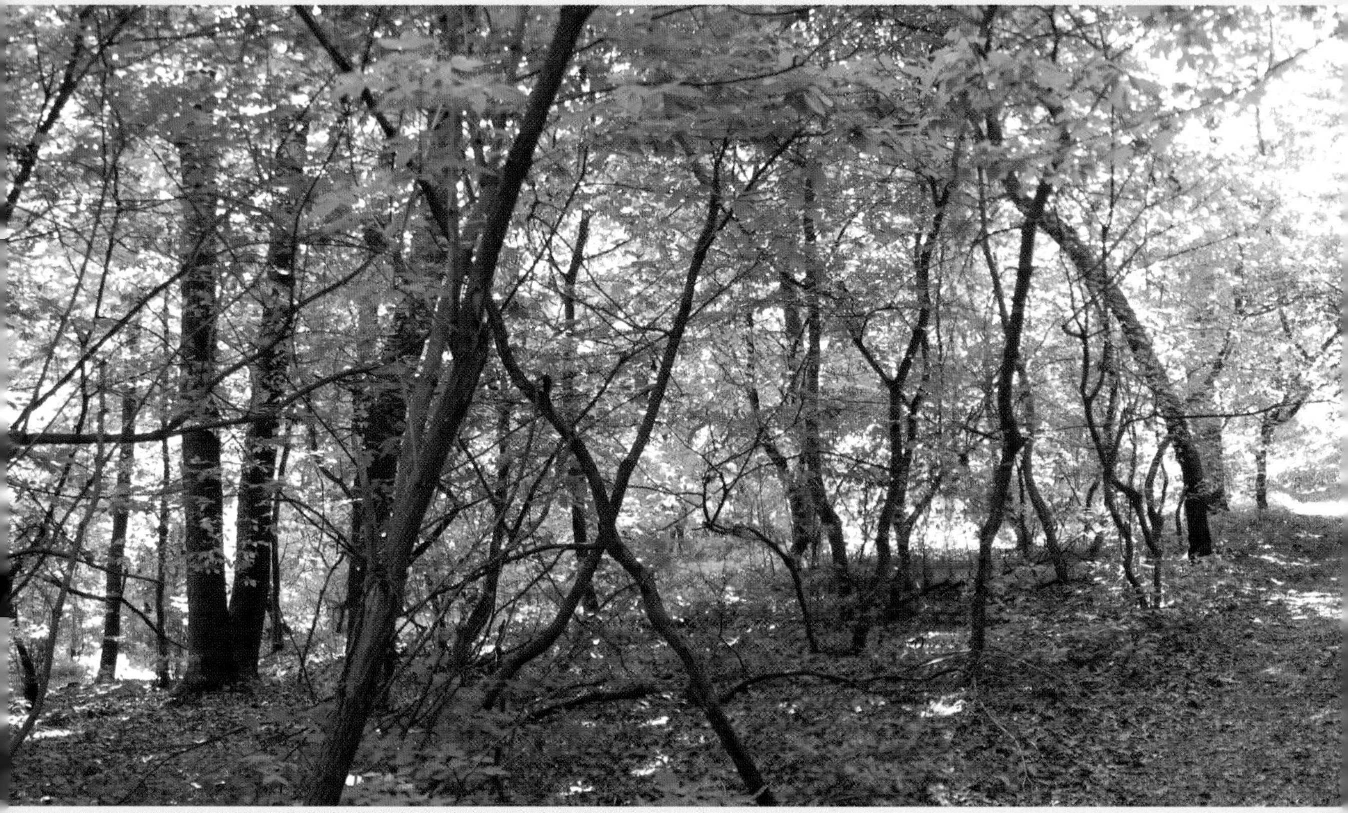

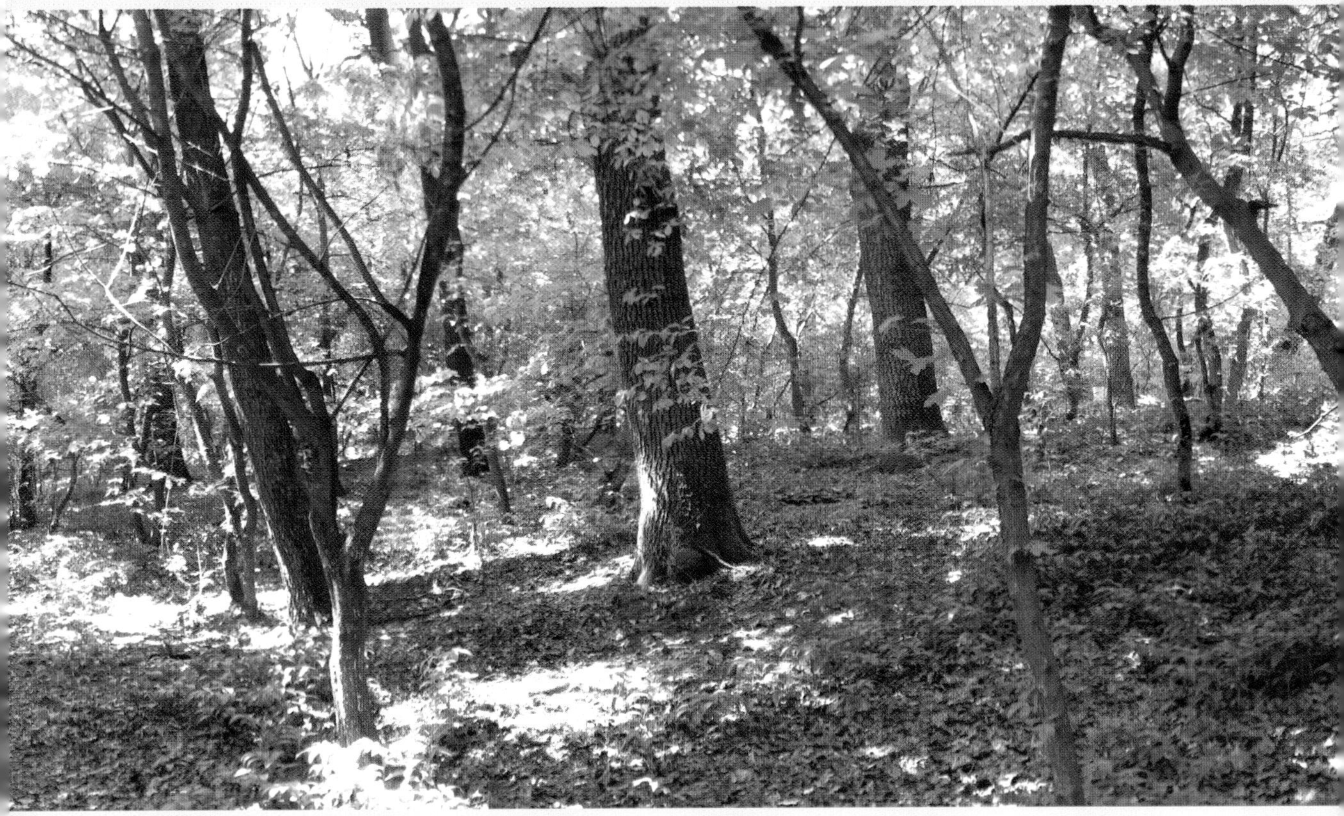

Contents

Introduction

The earth is a dynamic, living planet and, as far as we know, the only one that exists in this state. It is the photosynthesizing plants and their root microbes that make the earth different from all other planets. Much controversy has surrounded the subject of the creation of this planet and the solar system in which it resides. However, there are many fundamental aspects where most scientists can agree. The establishment of micro-organisms in the soil and water are essential to the survival of plants and other life forms. These microbes convert both organic and inorganic substances into carbon dioxide and elements that serve as a food source for plants.

Plants have the unique ability to absorb carbon dioxide from the atmosphere. In the presence of sunlight and water, plants also convert the sun's radiant energy to another form of potential energy – carbohydrates, starches and sugars – and then other complex chemicals in the process known as photosynthesis. Oxygen and water vapour are released back into the atmosphere as by-products of the molecular reactions in green plants. It is the photosynthetic process of plants that provides the earth with its oxygen-enriched environment that supports life on earth.

Plants and their photosynthetic processes have played an essential role in creating the gaseous atmosphere surrounding the planet. Only after plants and microbes were well established, was the planet inhabitable for all other life forms. These evolutionary events are important to understand. Also, plants in their abundance and the fruits they yield provide a ready supply of food, medicine and other beneficial products for animals and humans. We are dependent upon the microbial plant world for our existence and perhaps it is helpful to occasionally remind ourselves of this fact.

Plants play an important role in balancing the earth's ecosystems. Plants act as the 'lungs' of the earth by giving off oxygen and taking in carbon dioxide. In these processes, they also purify the air by removing airborne chemicals and pollutants. Marsh and wetland plants act as the 'kidneys' of the earth by removing toxic chemicals and other impurities from water.

We have known and understood these functions of plants for many years. As often is the case in science, however, an innovative new concept for improving indoor air quality (IAQ) came from an unlikely source. It took scientists at the US National Aeronautics and Space Administration (NASA) to discover how plants could purify and revitalize the air in the indoor environment. Their studies into ways of making long-term space habitation possible caused their scientists to rethink the processes that make earth inhabitable. In doing so, the concept of using plants to treat and recycle both air and water in the indoor environment was formed. After years of studies by scientists from around the world, the air and water cleansing functions of plants are more readily understood and these concepts are now gaining popularity. Constructed wetlands for treating both domestic and industrial wastewaters are now an accepted treatment method and are employed throughout the world. Innovative architects and builders have begun to view buildings as having their own micro-environment or micro-climate and have sought a more holistic approach to the maintenance and operation of buildings.

Although progress has been slow, many now see plant-human interaction within the confines of built spaces as having an important role in both the psychological and physiological well-being of its inhabitants. Many realize that plants are often placed within buildings merely for their aesthetic benefits: to soften hard surfaces and to provide ambience. Yet, scientific studies are now revealing the crucial need for humans to have consistent interaction with plants to produce optimal health and well-being. We now know that just viewing plants can reduce blood pressure and relieve stress. Studies have also shown that patients heal faster when plants are in view. Based on these findings, a new profession called 'horticultural therapy' has begun, devoted to the therapeutic value plants demonstrate in their relationship with humans. Other studies reveal that worker productivity increases and the number of sick leave decreases when plants are present in the work environment. These are important discoveries as those in industrialized nations often spend up to 90 per cent of their time indoors.

Since the beginning of civilization, people have used plants for medicinal purposes. Throughout history, people have held the belief that plants possess healing powers. The World Health Organization (WHO) estimates that up to 80 per cent of the world's population still relies mainly on herbal medicine for primary healthcare. This is especially true in developing nations and countries that have rainforests. It is predominantly the Western nations where medicines have transitioned from plant-derived prescriptions to synthetic ones. Today, only about 20 per cent of prescribed medicines in the US contain plant-derived chemicals.

The two primary methods of using plants for medicinal purpose are herbology and aromatherapy. Plants used as medicine, food seasonings and flavourings are known as herbs. Aromatherapy is the use of essential oils found in plants to enhance human health and well-being. Knowing that a plant has been used for a specific purpose for many years is an important clue in helping scientists target which plants might have medicinal value. In fact, indigenous people originally discovered the medicinal uses of three-quarters of the plant-derived medicines in use today.

As overwhelming evidence shows, synthetic prescriptions are often accompanied by a host of harmful side effects, many producing symptoms worse than the diseases they were meant to treat. As a result, there has been an explosive growth in the nutritional supplement market and herbal medicines are again becoming popular in Western countries.

However, it seems that just as modern science is beginning to rediscover the importance of herbal medicines, we are losing much of the earth's biological diversity. Most of the earth's plant diversity is found in rainforests. Rainforests once covered 14 per cent of the earth's land surface, but today they only cover 6 per cent. Yet, 50 to 90 per cent of the world's species diversity is found in the tropical regions. One hectare (2.47 acres) may contain more than 750 types of trees and 1,500 species of higher plants. As the rainforests disappear due to human encroachment, so do many possible cures for diseases. Thus far, less than 1 per cent of tropical trees and plants have been tested for their medicinal properties. For this reason alone, protection of the tropical rainforests is vital for humankind.

Throughout history, man has depended upon plants or the fruits and vegetables they yield for survival. Plants are rich in nutrients and phytochemicals that provide the human body with the essentials for nourishment and growth. From early recorded history man has cultivated plants for human sustenance. Today, however, man pursues the age-old practice of gardening essentially for the visual pleasure that foliage and ornamental plants provide. Few individuals in industrialized nations grow food for their own survival as food is readily available in nearby markets. Nevertheless, a growing number of people have come to realize that commercial farming operations yield crops containing fewer nutrients because of the use of synthetic fertilizers and are often laden with toxic pesticides. As a result, organic gardening and organic commercial farming are among the fastest growing segments in agriculture. Produce that is certified as organic is guaranteed to be free of harmful pesticides. It is expected that as more people become concerned about exposure to synthetic chemicals, the demand for organic products will continue to grow.

For thousands of years, primarily in Asian countries, plant ecosystems produced food by using human and animal waste as natural fertilizers. This process was not only a sustainable farming method but also prevented human and animal waste from polluting rivers and streams. For this reason, the waterways were less polluted than those in Western countries. These practices closely mimic what naturally occurs in nature in that these fertilizers provide all the nutritional elements necessary for optimal plant growth. However, the spreading of excrement on the topsoil is not hygienic and produces offensive odours. Due to the unsanitary nature of this method, it is now practised less. Many developing countries are transitioning to the Western method of synthetic, commercial fertilizers. However, synthetic fertilizers do not provide all the necessary trace elements and plants rapidly deplete them from the soil. In order to feed the world's burgeoning population, sustainable farming methods must be employed, albeit in a more hygienic manner.

By using hydroponic growing techniques, sustainable farming can be employed to produce crops by stripping wastewater of its nutrients. In this manner, we benefit both from the crop yield and the protection of our sensitive waterways. We have long understood that plant ecosystems function as the earth's 'kidneys' by filtering nutrients and pollutants from water. From expansive wetlands to small urban green spaces, each has the capacity to help filter impurities from the water passing through its ecosystem.

In many urban areas today, there is a concerted effort to incorporate the treatment of storm water runoff through green spaces. These 'eco-landscaping' methods are making great strides toward cleaning the water of its impurities before it winds its way into surrounding waterways. These efforts have also led architects and builders to view the roofs of buildings as an additional space for an oasis of green space in our crowded cities. Many roof gardens now help to filter water and slowly release the unused portion into the city's drainage system.

This book seeks to remind us all of our dependence on and interwoven connection with plants and their ecosystems. From the very air we breathe to the purity of the life-sustaining water we drink, plants play an integral role in our survival. In this post-modern era, we have again begun to recognize how our interactions with the plant world are vital for our health and well-being. As a result, more and more people seek to make this connection by growing plants within their own living spaces, both indoors and outdoors and by visiting public spaces such as national forests, public gardens, arboretums and extensive plantings within built spaces. No matter where we go to make a connection with plants, we are apt to benefit from the exposure. As more people make the connection between plants and human health, ecology gardens are destined to play a major role in our lives. Regardless of economic standing, almost everyone can experience nature at its best and the benefits to human health are significant.

Many people are aware of an inherent need to connect to the plant kingdom. Yet, in our hurried lifestyle we are often too busy 'to stop and smell the roses'. It is our hope that this book will provide the impetus for you to once again enjoy a connection with plants and their ecosystems and to understand just how vital plant ecosystems are to our survival.

Is the Air Indoors Making You Sick?

As energy consumption and its costs continue to rise, builders strive to tightly seal buildings to make them more energy-efficient. According to the US Department of Energy and the US Green Building Council, commercial and residential buildings use more than 60 per cent of all the electricity consumed in the US.

During the energy crisis of the 1970s, engineers began to seal building envelopes more tightly to conserve energy. A building envelope is the skin of the building that prevents air, moisture and heat from flowing in or out freely. It consists of exterior walls, windows, doors, floors and roofs. Almost immediately upon closing building envelopes, indoor air quality (IAQ) issues were raised by their inhabitants. Most building materials and furnishings today consist of synthetic materials that continuously release (or off-gas) gaseous chemicals into the indoor environment where they are trapped and become more concentrated.

In 1989, the US Environmental Protection Agency (EPA) submitted a report to the Congress on the quality of air found inside public buildings, including offices, hospitals, nursing homes and schools. This report stated that more than 900 volatile organic chemicals (VOCs) were identified that may pose serious acute and chronic health problems to individuals who live and work inside these buildings. Ten of these VOCs are listed in Table 1.1.

TABLE 1.1
SOME OF THE MORE THAN 900 VOCs FOUND IN THE AIR OF PUBLIC BUILDINGS

Benzene	Decane
Ethylbenzene	**FORMALDEHYDE**
Xylene	1,1,1-Trichloroethane
Styrene	Dichlorobenzene
Trichloroethylene	Ethyl Toluene

According to the US census in August 2000, fifty-four million households, or 51 per cent, had one or more computers. Nearly two-thirds (65 per cent) of all children aged three to seventeen years lived in a household with a computer in 2000. In 2001, engineers at the University of Texas conducted a study of the emissions of VOCs from personal computers. Some of these chemicals are shown in Table 1.2.

TABLE 1.2
CHEMICAL EMISSIONS FROM PERSONAL COMPUTERS

Toluene
Styrene
Dodecane
Benzaldehyde
Undecane
Butyraldehyde
Xylene
Ethyl benzene
Decane
1,2,4-Trimethylcyclohexane

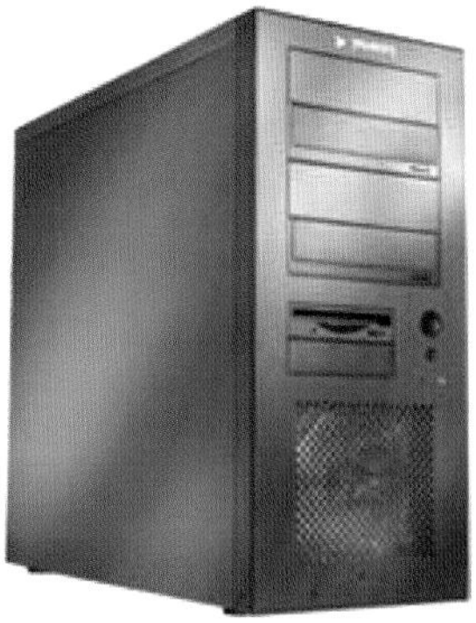

In a 1990 survey of computer monitors manufactured by IBM, researchers produced a listing of VOC emissions. Forty VOCs were identified. The ten leading hydrocarbon solvents are listed in Table 1.3.

Test chamber studies of ten television sets identified eighteen chemical emissions. Ten of those VOCs are listed in Table 1.4.

TABLE 1.3
CHEMICAL EMISSIONS FROM COMPUTER MONITORS

Toluene	Trimethylbenzene
Nonane	2-Ethoxyethyl Acetate
Xylene	Decane
Ethyl Benzene	Undecane
Styrene	Dodecane

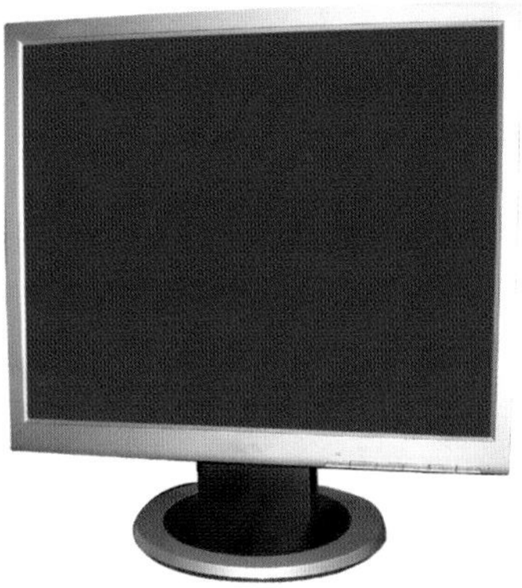

Studies have identified the indoor use of pesticides as a possible contributing factor in the growing number of brain tumours in small children. A study released in May 2000 by the researchers of Stanford University Medical School (USA) found that people who were exposed to pesticides at home were twice as likely to develop Parkinson's disease compared to those who were not exposed. Also, in 2000, Italian research physicians reported that exposure to hydrocarbon solvents found in common petroleum-based products, such as paints and glues, is a risk

TABLE 1.4
CHEMICAL EMISSIONS FROM TELEVISIONS

Benzene	Trichloroethene
Xylene	Tetrachloroethene
Styrene	2-butoxyethanol
Formaldehyde	Dibutylphthalate

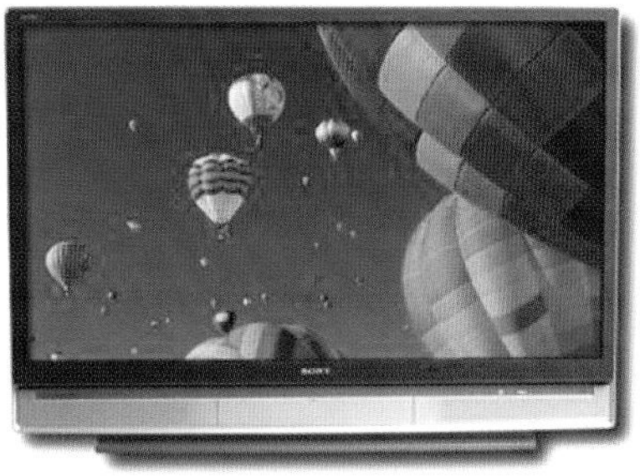

for an early onset of Parkinson's disease and increases the severity of the disease throughout its course.

In a benchmark study released by Environmental Working Group (July 2005), researchers found an average of 200 industrial chemical pollutants, including seven pesticides, in the umbilical cord blood of newborns. Of the chemicals detected, seventy-six were suspected of contributing to cancer in animals and humans, ninety-four are toxic to the brain and nervous system and seventy-nine can cause birth defects or abnormal development in animals. In 2003, EPA updated its cancer risk guidelines on finding that carcinogens (cancer-causing substances) are ten times as potent in babies and that some chemicals are up to sixty-five times more powerful in children, due primarily to their high rate of metabolism.

Asthma is defined as a chronic lung disease characterized by inflammation of the airways due to increased sensitivity to a variety of triggers, which can cause narrowing of the airways and breathing difficulty. Asthma currently affects more than twelve million Americans. There has been an alarming 74 per cent increase of asthma between 1980 and 1994 and children under the age of five have experienced an increase of 160 per cent. A recent study published in the British Medical Association's journal, *Thorax*, found that children exposed to higher levels of VOCs were four times more likely to suffer from asthma than children who were not.

However, increased cases of asthma are not limited to the US. The Global Burden of Asthma Report (May 2004) is a comprehensive survey of the prevalence and impact of asthma around the world, based on standardized data collected in epidemiology studies in more than eighty countries. According to this study, asthma is now one of the world's most common long-term conditions. The disease is estimated to affect as many as 300 million people worldwide.

Today, nearly forty-four million people in the East Asia/Pacific region have asthma. In

Taiwan, asthma symptoms have increased almost five-fold over a twenty-year period. In Japan, the number of asthma patients treated by medical facilities today is over 100 cases per 100,000 people. However, just thirty years ago, the rate was three cases per 100,000. In Oceania (Australia, New Zealand and the Pacific Islands), the prevalence of asthma is about 15 per cent, making it among the highest in the world. In China and India, the current rate of asthma is only 2 per cent and 3.5 per cent, respectively. However, due to population density, this amounts to about 27.8 million people in China and approximately 35 million in India. As these countries surge toward urbanization, these trends are predicted to rise sharply in the next decade.

Another common malady associated with indoor air quality issues is multiple chemical sensitivity (MCS). MCS is a syndrome in which multiple symptoms occur with low-level chemical exposure. Currently, there is insufficient scientific evidence to establish a relationship between the causes and the symptoms. However, the possible causes are allergy, toxic effects and neurological sensitivity. There have been few studies on the synergistic effects caused by exposure to low levels of multiple chemicals.

The term sick building syndrome (SBS) is used to describe a range of symptoms experienced by a high proportion of those living and working in a particular building or part of a building. Standard analysis can detect no cause or origin for their illness. When the building occupants are away for a given time, the symptoms usually diminish, only to recur upon re-entry into the building. Symptoms commonly associated with SBS are: allergies; eye, nose and throat irritations; fatigue; headache; nervous system disorders; respiratory congestion and sinus congestion.

The term building related illness (BRI) is used to describe diseases that can be attributed directly to airborne building contaminants. Examples of BRI include lung cancer contracted from asbestos exposure and legionnaire's disease caused by bacteria in stagnant water in air conditioning or heating systems.

With all these findings, it should not be surprising that EPA now ranks indoor air pollution among the top five threats to human health. The costs associated with poor indoor air quality are staggering as well. In 2000, researchers William T. Fisk and Arthur H. Rosenfeld, Lawrence Berkeley National Laboratory (US), found that American companies could save $58 billion annually by preventing SBS and an additional $200 billion in improved worker productivity due to better IAQ. The same study verified that 40 per cent of all sick days are IAQ-related.

When adjusted for inflation, these costs would be even greater today.

CAUSES OF SICK BUILDING/ HOUSE SYNDROME

Ventilation

Ventilation is the introduction of outside air into a building, primarily through forced air movement by mechanical means. Its goal is to improve IAQ by diluting the stale indoor air created by human respiration with fresh outside air. With each breath we take, we not only emit carbon dioxide (CO_2) but also hundreds of trace levels of VOCs. The human body is a living biological machine which emits many different chemicals that can cause stale air to build up, especially in crowded rooms. The VOCs emitted by the human body and respiratory system are called bio-effluents. So, the more heavily a building is populated, the greater the bio-effluents emitted into the indoor environment. Today, there are hundreds of VOCs emitted by synthetic products found in homes, offices and other buildings. When these VOCs are combined with bio-effluents in tightly sealed, energy-efficient buildings, indoor air pollution becomes a serious health threat. Because humans emit sufficient quantities of CO_2 to be easily monitored, CO_2 is commonly used as an indicator of polluted, stale air. Carbon dioxide does not present a health problem even at several thousand parts per million. It is the combination of CO_2, VOCs, microbes, etc., that is of concern.

Most buildings bring in fresh air through an outside duct and mix it with re-circulated air. The presumption made is that the outside air is clean. However, this is often not the case, especially in urban or industrialized areas. Ventilation is only one component of a building's HVAC (heating, ventilation and air conditioning) system.

As a result of the 1973 oil embargo, ventilation was reduced to 0.14 cubic m (5 cfm) per minute of outside air for each building occupant in a national energy conservation move. It quickly became apparent that this was inadequate. In an effort to combat IAQ problems, the American Society of Heating, Refrigerating and Air Conditioning Engineers (ASHRAE) has continually recommended increasing ventilation rates in an effort to purge the air. However, this approach during the past thirty years has failed to solve the problem. Ventilation has four inherent problems: 1) Reduced energy efficiency; 2) An assumption of clean outside air; 3) Controlling the temperature variation between outside and inside air; and 4) Increased vulnerability to bioterrorism.

The sole purpose of energy-efficient buildings is to reduce energy consumption.

Opening a building's envelope through increased ventilation defeats the purpose of energy conservation. Many buildings' IAQ problems are due to design and operational flaws. Poor placement of ventilation ducts and improperly maintained HVAC systems are leading IAQ issues. A study by the Healthy Building Institute found that only 38 per cent of the 1,136 major buildings inspected were well ventilated with efficiently filtered air-handling units and clean, well-maintained ventilation systems.

March 1995 brought a new reality to the civilized world when an extremist group released the nerve agent Sarin into the Tokyo subway system. The attack killed twelve and injured more than 5,000. Until 11 September 2001, few had given much thought regarding the vulnerability of ventilation systems to biological agents. Though thousands were killed in New York City at ground zero, many more may now be suffering chronic respiratory problems from breathing the toxic dust and chemical vapours that entered schools and other nearby buildings through air ducts after the twin towers collapsed.

A biological/chemical attack would be devastating to a massive number of people and produce severe economic consequences. The most likely approach terrorists might use is to employ an aerosolizer to release biological or chemical warfare agents into a building's ventilation ducts. Currently, no reliable means exist for detecting biological agents released into the atmosphere. Agents would probably go unrecognized until building occupants begin to exhibit symptoms. Today, most buildings use only dust filters without 'treating' the outside air, primarily because it is cost-prohibitive. Even if cost was not an issue, high-efficiency particulate arrester (HEPA) filters cannot filter chemical agents. They do have the ability to trap biological agents, but cannot destroy them. Some buildings use standard gaseous adsorbent media, such as treated activated carbon, to trap chemical pollutants. Once the HEPA filter or gaseous adsorbent media has been saturated with pathogenic microbes and/or toxic chemicals, the issue becomes one of safe disposal. If saturated filters or filtering media are not changed immediately, they begin to release the chemical back into the building. Clearly, the realities of life in the twenty-first century call for new considerations about the vulnerabilities posed by building ventilation.

Chemical Emissions

Among the top contributors to indoor air pollution are chemicals that off-gas from many of the products used to construct, furnish, operate and maintain buildings. During the last several decades, the building industry has experienced a significant change in the composition of building materials and furnishings. Prior to that, natural wood or plant fibres were used in construction, whereas now, pressed wood products or fibreboard are predominantly used. Wall-to-wall carpeting is now the most common floor covering. Home and office furnishings primarily comprise synthetic materials held together with a variety of glues and resins.

Before the twentieth century, man-made chemicals were virtually unknown. Today, there are more than 80,000 synthetic chemicals in use and, alarmingly, there is no toxicity data on four out of five of these. New synthetic materials and furnishings commonly emit or off-gas chemicals. The rate at which chemicals are emitted varies. Generally speaking, emissions are highest when products are new but may continue at lower rates for a number of years. Factors such as temperature and humidity also influence the rate of emissions. As the temperature and/or humidity rise, emissions increase.

The EPA found that VOC levels may be ten to thousands of times higher indoors than outdoors. A single indoor air sample may commonly contain from fifty to hundreds of VOCs. The few toxicity studies that have been conducted focused on a single chemical or chemical compound and at relatively high concentration levels. Little, if any, studies have examined the synergistic effects possible from a mixture of chemicals emitted in low concentrations. Therefore, no one can say definitively what the short- or long-term health effects might be on the human population living and working in buildings whose air comprises a 'chemical soup' of synthetic emissions. Table 1.5 lists some common sources of VOCs.

Formaldehyde

Formaldehyde is one of the leading chemical compounds in indoor air emissions. It is a common industrial chemical used to make other chemicals, building materials and household products. It is a component of many of the following products:

- Pressed wood products (particleboard, hardwood plywood and fibreboard)
- Urea-formaldehyde foam insulation
- Paper products
- Some paints, stains and varnishes
- Permanent press clothing, draperies and upholstery

(See Table 1.5 for a comprehensive listing.)

Formaldehyde is a colourless gas with a pungent, irritating odour. It is the most commonly found indoor air pollutant. It can produce several symptoms, including watery eyes, burning sensation in the eyes, nose and throat, headaches and fatigue. At higher concentrations, people may experience upper

TABLE 1.5 SOURCES OF CHEMICAL EMISSIONS	Formaldehyde	Xylene/Toluene	Benzene	Trichloroethylene	Chloroform	Ammonia	Alcohols	Acetone
Adhesives	•	•	•				•	
Bio-effluents		•				•	•	•
Blueprint machines						•		
Carpeting*	•						•	
Caulking compounds	•	•	•				•	
Ceiling tiles	•	•	•				•	
Chlorinated tap water					•			
Cleaning products						•		
Cosmetics							•	•
Duplicating machines				•				
Electrophotographic printers		•	•	•		•		
Draperies	•							
Fabrics	•							
Facial tissues	•							
Floor coverings	•	•	•				•	
Gas stoves	•							
Grocery bags	•							
Microfiche developers						•		
Nail polish remover								•
Office correction fluid								•
Paints	•	•	•				•	
Paper towels	•							
Particleboard	•	•	•				•	
Permanent-press clothing	•							
Photocopiers		•	•	•		•		
Plywood	•							
Pre-printed paper forms								•
Stains and varnishes	•	•	•				•	
Tobacco smoke	•		•					
Upholstery	•							
Wall coverings		•	•				•	

* New carpets do not normally contain formaldehyde. However, they may trap formaldehyde emitted from other sources and later release the formaldehyde into the indoor air whenever the humidity and temperature change.

and lower respiratory irritation resulting in difficulty in breathing and it may even trigger attacks in asthma patients. Formaldehyde is listed as a human carcinogen by the US government. Extended inhalation is expected to increase the incidence of symptoms. Children, the elderly, and those with compromised immune symptoms are most vulnerable to formaldehyde exposure.

In the fall of 2005, the US Federal Emergency Management Association (FEMA) distributed an estimated 150,000 travel trailers and mobile homes to people in Mississippi, Louisiana, Alabama, Texas and Florida, who had lost their homes in Hurricanes Katrina and Rita. The high surface-to-volume ratio of particleboard and plywood used in travel trailers, as well as lower air-exchange rates, are the primary causes of formaldehyde concentrations. Responding to the numerous complaints voiced by residents of the FEMA trailers, a local Sierra Club began conducting numerous indoor air quality tests. They found unsafe levels of formaldehyde in thirty out of the thirty-two trailers tested.

Unfortunately, finding a responsible federal agency willing to take action has been nearly impossible. In February 2007, representative Gene Taylor (D-Mississippi) wrote a letter to the Centers for Disease Control and Prevention (CDC) urging a 'detailed investigation' into formaldehyde levels in the travel trailers provided by FEMA. However, the CDC's 29 May response only served to point out a bewildering maze of federal bureaucracy. So, four years after the devastating 2005 hurricane season, thousands continue to not only struggle to rebuild their lives but are suffering various physical ailments due to conditions inside their temporary housing. In August 2007, FEMA reversed its course and ordered the CDC to conduct air quality tests. FEMA also agreed to move those complaining of health problems out of the travel trailers and into more permanent housing.

The indoor air pollution problem is not limited to FEMA trailers. High levels of formaldehyde may be more common in all types of travel trailers, RVs (recreational vehicles) and mobile homes. These homes are constructed primarily with pressed wood products. They are often left closed for extended periods of time and have little ventilation to purge the formaldehyde-laden air. The Sierra Club also tested thirteen different types of RVs used as FEMA trailers and all models had some tests showing elevated levels of formaldehyde (see Chapter Two, page 48 for additional information on formaldehyde removal in FEMA trailers).

According to an article on 8 October 2006 in the *Los Angeles Times*, 'cargo shiploads of birch and poplar plywood are arriving in

California carrying two labels: one proclaiming "Made in China" while the other warns that it contains formaldehyde.' This plywood is commonly used in the manufacture of kitchen cabinets, appliance cabinets, furniture, including bunk beds and other products in mobile homes and standard built homes. In 2005 alone, China exported to the US more than half a billion dollars' worth of hardwood plywood – enough to build cabinets for two million kitchens. Much of the plywood, fibreboard and particleboard sold in the US is manufactured with adhesives or glues that contain formaldehyde. Many countries in the European Union, Japan, China and others have more stringent environmental standards that ban these products. However, it remains legal in the US.

The article further states that 'one birch plank from China, bought at a Home Depot in Portland, gave off 100 times more formaldehyde than is legal in Japan and 30 times more than is allowed in Europe and China'. This is especially troubling since low-cost, chemical-free substitutes are available. Columbia Forest Products is one of the few US companies to make the switch to non-toxic glues made of soy flour.

More recently a 17 March 2009 article in *USA Today* states that possibly tens of thousands of homes in Florida, Virginia, Alabama and other southern states contain Chinese imported drywall. Drywall is the board used to make interior walls in many buildings. Some of these drywalls emit sulphides that are very corrosive to copper coils, electronics and plumbing components. These gaseous sulphides have a rotten egg odour. Until federal regulations are made more stringent in the US, the American public cannot reasonably expect to significantly lower its exposure to formaldehyde, sulphides or other potentially harmful products.

Biological Contaminants

Biological contaminants consist of bacteria, moulds, mildew, viruses, dust mites, cockroaches, animal dander and pollen. Bacteria are commonly found in ventilation and cooling systems and in deposits of dust and dirt. As bacteria disintegrate or decompose, they may release endotoxins. Endotoxins present human health problems whenever they become aerosolized as dust particles. By breathing in these dust particles, the endotoxins can penetrate deeply into the lungs, causing respiratory discomfort.

Many biological contaminants, such as moulds and mildew, require warm, damp environments to thrive. Standing water, water-damaged materials and wet surfaces are all excellent breeding grounds. In fact, any time a surface remains wet for more than forty-eight hours mould growth is likely to occur. Careful attention to maintenance and regulating relative humidity levels between 30 to 50 per cent can greatly minimize the presence of these contaminants.

Pollen originates from plants, is most often seasonal, and is primarily introduced into the indoor environment through ventilation systems. Inhalation of pollen can trigger allergic responses, hay fever and asthma. Pollen counts are highest usually during the spring and summer months. Most interior plants are foliage plants that do not produce flowers or pollen.

Humans and animals transmit viruses. Infectious diseases such as influenza, measles, tuberculosis and chicken pox are transmitted through the air. Household pets are sources of saliva and animal dander. The protein in urine from rats and mice is a potent allergen. When it dries, it can become airborne. Household dust mites are often contributors to allergies. Dust mites live in fabrics, carpets, pillows and mattresses. Removal of carpeting can greatly reduce the presence of dust mites. Dust mites can be further reduced, though not eliminated altogether, by a regimen of thorough cleaning.

FILTRATION TECHNOLOGY

There are a variety of conventional methods that are currently used to filter indoor air. The three most common ones are HEPA filters, gaseous adsorbents, such as activated carbon and zeolite, and ultraviolet light.

HEPA Filters

High-efficiency particulate arrester (HEPA) filters were originally designed to remove and capture radioactive dust particles from air to prevent health hazards to the personnel working at the Atomic Energy Commission laboratory. These devices filter and retain all particles from the air that passes through them, starting from 0.3 microns in size at an efficiency rating of 99.97 per cent. HEPA filters comprise paper-like materials made of very thin glass fibres that provide pleats to increase the surface area.

Powerful fan motors are required to force air through the small holes. Filter holes physically trap the particles thereby removing them from indoor air. Therefore, efficiency is greatly reduced over time and the filters must be replaced. Their use is generally restricted to small systems, primarily due to fan noise. With proper maintenance and filter replacement, HEPA filters are highly efficient in removing particles and microbes larger than 0.3 microns from indoor air. But these larger microbes are only trapped, not destroyed. As a result, the filter becomes a breeding ground for trapped microbes. Therefore, timely replacement of filters is imperative. Unfortunately, many find regular filter replacement cost-prohibitive. Most viruses are smaller than 0.3 microns and are not trapped by the HEPA filter. Also, HEPA filters are not designed to remove VOCs and, therefore, do nothing to combat one of the major IAQ problems.

Activated Carbon Filters

Activated carbon filters have been used for many years to remove VOCs from the air. Activated carbon is a porous, sponge-like substance that can collect and retain certain chemical compounds on its surface. The surface of activated carbon is very large, ranging from 9,684 to 13,988 square feet (900 to 1,300 sq m) per gram of carbon. Activated carbon is manufactured by burning wood, coconut shell, coal or other substances at 800-1000°C (1,472-1,832°F) in a controlled atmosphere, producing millions of sub-microscopic holes in the carbon surface. There are many types and grades of activated carbon depending upon the raw material and the degree of activation.

The ability of activated carbon to remove VOCs from air is generally given as a per cent of its own weight to remove carbon tetrachloride. For example, 80 per cent 'adsorption capacity' means that one gram of activated carbon can remove 0.8 grams of carbon tetrachloride at 25°C (77°F). Some of the common compounds for which activated carbon has low adsorption capacity, especially at high relative humidity, are carbon monoxide, methane, ammonia, carbon dioxide, methylene chloride, nitrous oxide, formaldehyde and other small molecules. However, certain substances can be impregnated on carbon to increase their removal rates for otherwise poorly adsorbed chemicals, as is the case with gas mask filters.

One of the significant shortcomings of activated carbon filters and HEPA filters is that they trap chemicals but do not destroy them. Therefore, it is difficult to accurately predict when these filters become saturated and are no longer effective in removing hazardous materials from indoor air.

Zeolite

Zeolites are natural volcanic minerals with unique characteristics. Their chemical structure classifies them as hydrated aluminosilicates comprising hydrogen, oxygen, aluminium and silicon. The honeycomb structure of zeolite produces connecting channels that vary in size from 2.5 to 5.0 angstroms. Zeolite has the capacity to adsorb ammonia, hydrogen sulphide, formaldehyde and other small molecular weight chemicals that are poorly adsorbed by activated carbon. Therefore, a mixture of activated carbon and zeolite makes an excellent adsorptive medium for removing airborne chemicals.

Germicidal Ultraviolet (UV) light

UV light bulbs have been used for more than fifty years to reduce pathogenic microbes in the air of classrooms, operating rooms, nurseries, bacteriology laboratories, restaurants and other food establishments. UV light is lethal because it is absorbed by the cells' nucleic acids. When absorbed, cross-links in loops of a DNA strand are produced between neighbouring thymine molecules. These thymine dimers inhibit the normal replication of the DNA by blocking the passage of the replicating enzyme. The most effective UV light waves for killing microbes are 254-260 nanometres (nm) in length. Wavelengths below 250 nm may produce excessive amounts of ozone that also kill microbes. However, ozone at levels high enough to destroy microbes may also cause respiratory problems in some individuals.

Because UV light can cause inflammation if directed into the eyes, lamps are placed high on the walls with UV light directed toward the ceiling of the room, or placed in room air ducts or concealed inside filters. UV light bulbs need replacing every one to three years depending upon use.

There are other types of filters, mostly electronic, that are marketed as effective in improving indoor air quality but lack the many years of proof as is the case with HEPA, activated carbon and UV light.

SUMMARY

Indoor air quality is a serious human health issue having no single solution. Many of the problems associated with HVAC systems could be reduced or alleviated with a stricter, regimented approach to maintenance. Today, products are available that have lower chemical emissions and more such are coming into the market. The consumer can now require that products, such as carpeting, go through a period of time to allow for major off-gassing before installation. In many countries, it is becoming sociably unacceptable to use tobacco products in public spaces. While all of these efforts are helpful, remediation of indoor air pollution is yet to take place. Many VOCs are carcinogenic and some may contribute to the development of asthma. Therefore, new technologies are needed that can purify and revitalize indoor air while maintaining energy efficiency in tightly sealed buildings.

After years of failed conventional methods to alleviate indoor air pollution, perhaps it is now time to take a look at the benefits plant ecosystems might offer in the struggle for clean air in the indoor environment.

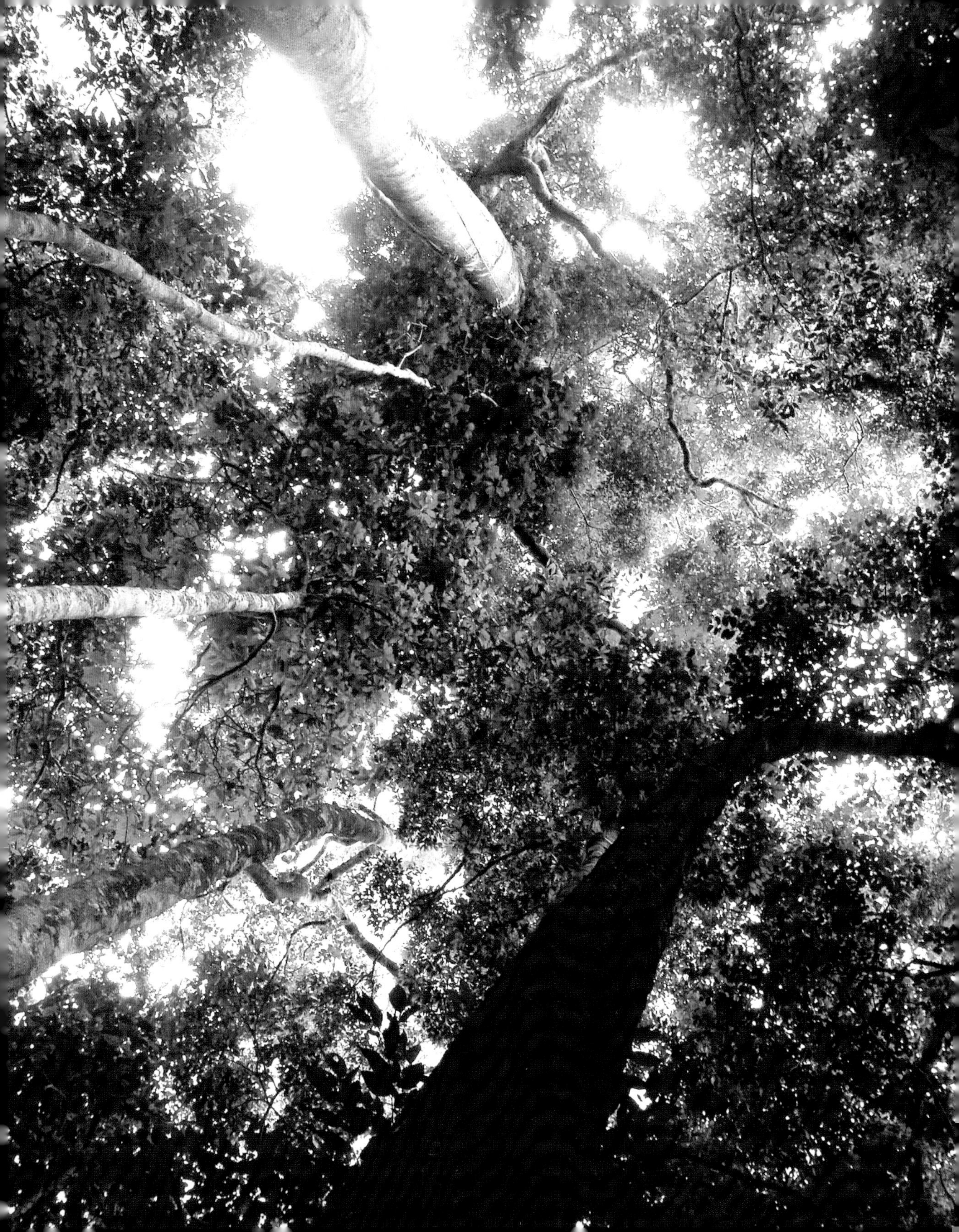

Plants: Nature's Air Purifiers

Scientists estimate that the earth is approximately 4.5 billion years old. Long ago, astronomers determined that the earth is a planet revolving around the sun in our solar system. Many other solar systems exist in the great beyond. Yet, as far as man can determine, earth is the only planet that sustains life. Why is that?

The first forms of life on earth were micro-organisms. Millions of years after the appearance of microbes, plants first appeared on earth. It is important to note that before plants could survive, micro-organisms had to become established in the earth's soil and water. Micro-organisms are essential to plants because they convert organic and inorganic substances into a form that is used by plants for food. The zone on earth in which life naturally occurs extends from the deep crust to the lower atmosphere. It is this area that is commonly referred to as the biosphere. It is the biosphere that makes earth a living, dynamic planet.

The oxygen produced during the photosynthetic process of plants is vital to all organisms that require it for respiration. This life-supporting oxygen is carried over earth's entire surface by wind currents. The living processes of animals and humans would deplete the atmosphere of oxygen if it were not replenished by photosynthesis.

Photosynthesis is not only essential for the maintenance of all higher forms of life, but is also a process of immense magnitude. An estimated 170 billion tons of dry plant biomass is produced through photosynthesis by all plants on earth each year. For every dry ton of new plant biomass produced through photosynthesis, approximately 1.4 tons (1,273 kg) of oxygen is added to the atmosphere and approximately 1.8 tons (1,636 kg) of carbon dioxide is removed. Tropical rainforests cover approximately 6 per cent of the earth's land surface, yet support up to 50 per cent of the world's life forms, estimated to be somewhere near

30 million plant, animal and insect species. With the earth's burgeoning population growth and the rate at which rainforests are being destroyed, one wonders just how long the world's plant ecosystems can continue to sustain life.

In 1772, English scientist Joseph Priestly discovered the ability of plants to purify air. He found that air in chambers made unclean by animal respiration and burning candles could be made pure again by plants. Dutch physician Jan Ingenhousz added to Priestly's discovery in 1778 by showing how light, striking green plant leaves improved air quality. We now know that this is made possible through the photosynthetic process. Like most living beings, plants use sugar for energy but they have the unique ability to manufacture their own sugar.

Photosynthesis can take place only in the presence of light. Plants absorb carbon dioxide from the atmosphere through tiny openings in their leaves called stomata. Plant roots absorb moisture from the soil. Chlorophyll and other green tissues in the leaves absorb radiant energy from a light source. This energy is used to split water molecules into oxygen and hydrogen. Through complex chemical reactions, plants use hydrogen and carbon dioxide to form sugars. Oxygen, a by-product of photosynthesis, is then released into the atmosphere.

In 1782, Swiss scientist Jean Senebier reported how the air-restoring activity of plants depends on the presence of carbon dioxide. In 1864, French plant physiologist T.B. Boussingault put photosynthesis on a quantitative basis and found that approximately equal volumes of oxygen were emitted and carbon dioxide absorbed during the process.

A varied population of micro-organisms lives in the soil. The rhizosphere (zone of soil influenced by plant roots) contains more microbes than other soil because of the

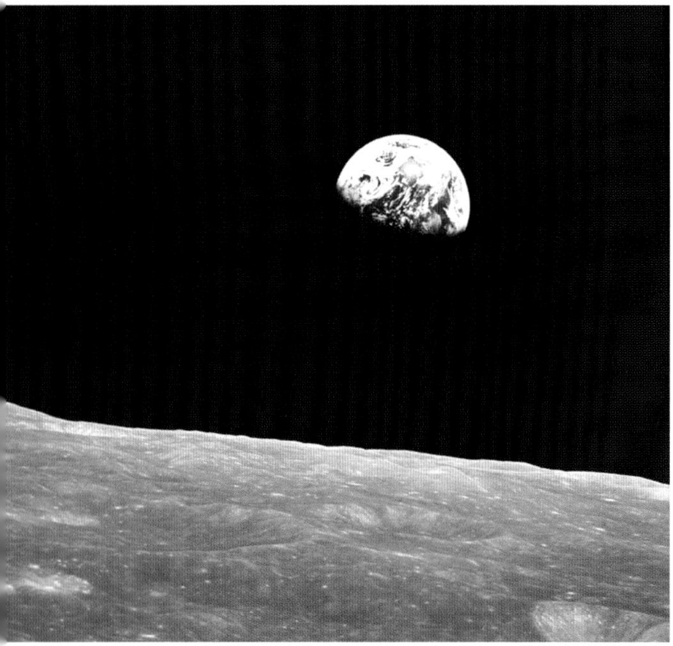

FIG. 2.1

availability of food. Organic compounds excreted from the roots or dead root cells serve as a food source for microbes. Certain bacteria commonly found in the rhizosphere of some plants can rapidly mutate and adapt, enhancing their ability to break down a variety of environmental pollutants. The synergistic reactions taking place between plants and their root microbes create one of nature's most powerful tools for cleaning air and water.

It is commonly understood that vegetation, especially the tropical rainforests, supplies the earth with oxygen-enriched air, making our survival possible. Children are taught the importance of rainforests and our need to preserve them at an early age. Yet, it seems difficult for our modern society to correlate that if we spend as much as 90 per cent of our time indoors, sealed away from nature, it is neither natural nor healthy. A building is basically a box filled with synthetic building materials and furnishings, electronic equipment and a vast assortment of supplies. Practically all items within a building release chemical vapours, producing, at any given moment, a mixture of vapours of unknown quantity or toxicity. To reduce energy costs, most building managers recycle the existing air and reduce the flow of outside air into the building. Little wonder that the air often becomes a stagnant, chemical soup.

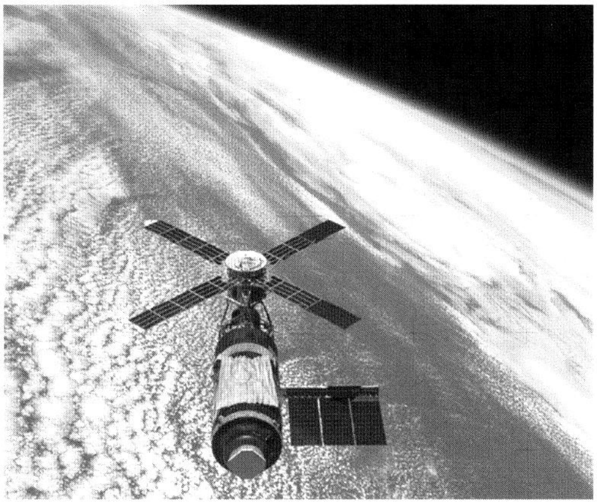

FIG. 2.2

The Biohome

In 1969, NASA accomplished one of man's greatest technological feats when it successfully landed astronauts on the moon. Looking back on the earth, NASA began to contemplate the possibilities of long-term space habitation. It soon became apparent that permanently manned habitats in outer space would need to closely mimic the earth's bio-regenerative processes. NASA sought to perfect a 'closed ecological life support system' integrating man's mechanical technology with nature's plant/microbial systems. During this plant research project, several applications for cleaning the environment were developed and are now being applied to help solve the earth's environmental pollution problems.

In a 1973 Skylab III mission, NASA detected the presence of more than 300

VOCs and identified 107 compounds in the air inside the spacecraft during occupancy by its crew. As a result of this mission, NASA realized that a tightly sealed structure primarily composed of synthetic materials could create serious indoor air quality issues through the outgassing (release) of VOCs.

In 1983, the EPA identified more than 350 VOCs inside an energy-efficient home for the elderly in Washington, DC. By 1988, EPA had identified more than 900 VOCs inside newly constructed public buildings. Coincidentally, between 1984 and 1994, asthma in American children had increased by an alarming rate of 160 per cent. Indoor air pollution is the leading suspect for this rapid increase.

In 1980, NASA scientists at the John C Stennis Space Center in Mississippi first discovered that interior plants could remove VOCs from sealed test chambers. After many repetitive chamber tests, NASA's findings were published in 1984. These findings were enthusiastically received by the public. Realizing its potential value, key leaders within the interior 'plantscape' and plant grower industries, including Gary Mangum, Gerry Leider, Don Horowitz, Dean Richardson, Tony Costa, Nan Hoback, Barbara Halfman and Joe Cialone, developed a keen interest

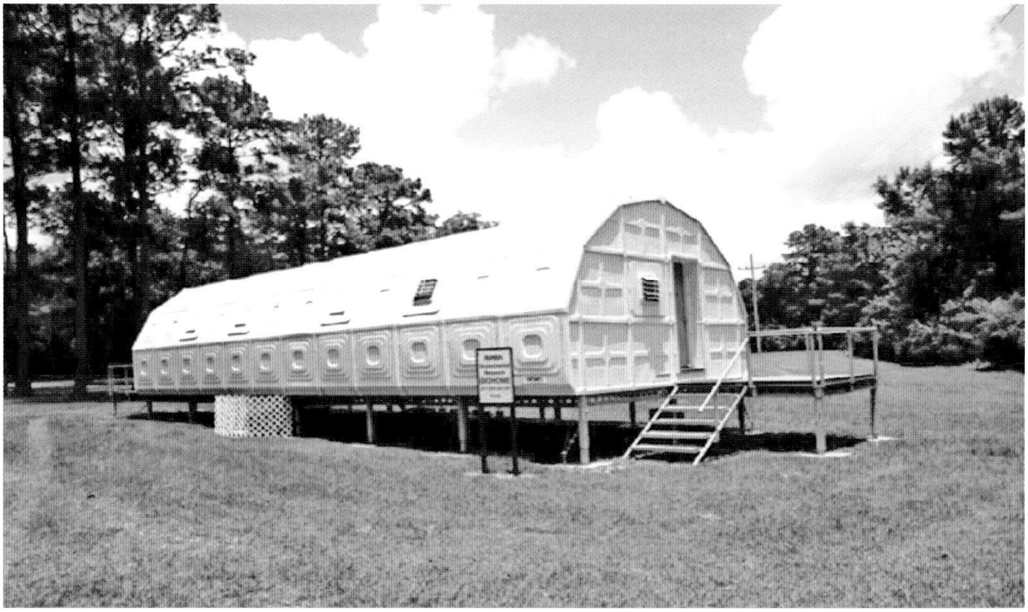

FIG. 2.3

in funding further research. As a result, the Associated Landscape Contractors of America (ALCA), which is now the Professional Landcare Network (PLANET), jointly funded a two-year study with NASA to further evaluate twelve common interior plants for their ability to remove three common airborne contaminants: formaldehyde, benzene and trichloroethylene from sealed test chambers.

This study produced additional results proving that interior plants can consistently remove airborne contaminants. Interestingly, it showed that some plants are more effective in their removal capacity than others. The results of this study were published in September 1989 and released in a press conference held at the National Press Club in Washington, DC. A non-profit organization, formerly known as the Plants for Clean Air Council, and later as Plants at Work, headed by Jan Roy, was established to mount a national information campaign working in conjunction with the industry to inform professionals and the public about the numerous benefits of interior plants. The organization, now headed by Media Director M.J. Gilhooley, has recently changed its name to Green Plants for Green Buildings. Their website address is www.greenplantsforgreenbuildings.org.

To further investigate these findings, NASA constructed a 'Biohome' made entirely of synthetic materials and engineered to achieve maximum air and energy closure. As shown in Fig. 2.3, its exterior consisted of moulded plastic panels designed to resist normal weather conditions with minimal maintenance. Fibreglass insulation in the walls (30 cm thickness) provided a thermal insulation value of R-40, making it super energy-efficient. The Biohome's dimensions are 43 ft (13.1 m) in length with 640 sq ft (59.5 sq m) of total interior space. The interior space is subdivided into a 334 sq ft (32 sq m) fully equipped, one-person habitat and a 306 sq ft (27.5 sq m) section housing bio-regenerative components, whose basic end products were reclaimed water and food.

The Biohome primarily comprised synthetic building materials and furnishings. Therefore, it was assumed that outgassing of VOCs would create indoor air quality problems. Upon entering the Biohome, the most exhibited symptoms were burning eyes and throat and respiratory problems.

Foliage plants that thrive in low-light conditions were placed throughout the living quarters to evaluate their ability to remove the VOCs built up from off-gassing of the newly constructed and furnished facility (Fig. 2.4). Scientists placed an array of interior plants growing in commercial potting soil throughout the Biohome. Additionally, they placed one experimental fan-assisted planter containing a

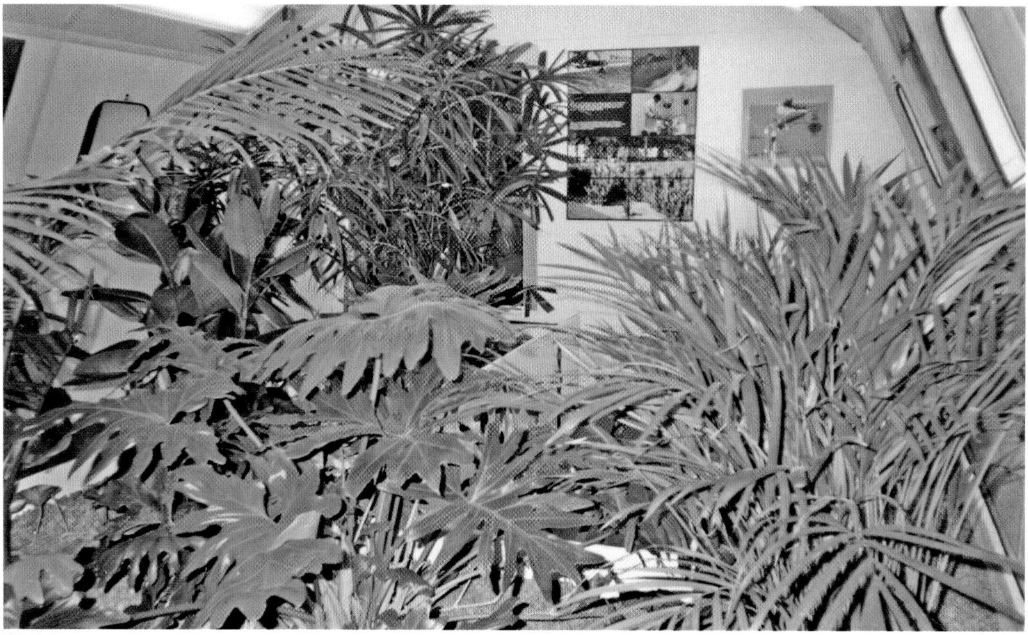

FIG. 2.4

plant growing in a mixture of soil and activated carbon (explained later in the chapter). This unique plant filter had the VOC removal capacity of fifteen regularly potted plants (Fig. 2.5).

Air quality was tested several days later by mass spectrometer/gas chromatograph analyses showing that nearly all of the VOCs had been removed (see Fig. 2.6).

Sophisticated chemical analyses are necessary for scientific validation. However, the definitive proof lay in the fact that one no longer experienced burning eyes or other classic symptoms of SBS when entering the Biohome. This was the first 'real world' application of interior plants for alleviating SBS. As a case study, a student lived for one summer in the Biohome and experienced no discomfort from indoor air quality (Fig. 2.7).

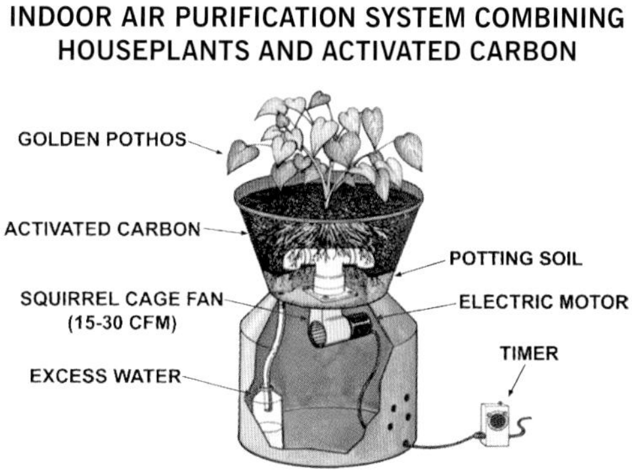

FIG. 2.5

After the research programme concluded, NASA moved the Biohome to the Visitor's Center and renamed it 'One Mainstreet Mars'. It continued its role as a valuable educational tool by simulating a life-support module on Mars where the air and waste are treated by interior plants. For many years, One Mainstreet Mars was one of the most popular exhibits for the young and old alike. Unfortunately, it was destroyed on 29 August 2005 by Hurricane Katrina.

Plants and their Microbes

Technology termed 'phytoremediation' utilizes plants and their root microbes to remove contaminants from both air and water. *Phyto* is the Greek word for plant and *remediation* is the process of correcting a problem or to put back in proper condition. During the early 1990s, studies sought to determine the mechanisms plant ecosystems utilize to remove VOCs from sealed chambers. The NASA studies employed only a one-time injection of VOCs into the test chambers. Questions arose whether plants could remove VOCs that were continuously off-gassed from synthetic materials as commonly occurs in an indoor environment.

To answer this issue, Wolverton Environmental Services, Inc. (WES)

COMPARISON OF CHEMICAL PRESENCE WITH AND WITHOUT PLANTS
(Gas Chromatograph/Mass Spectrometer Data, November 1987)

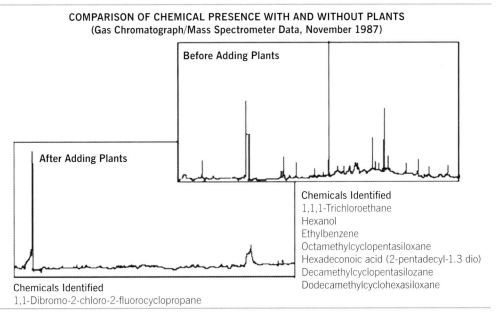

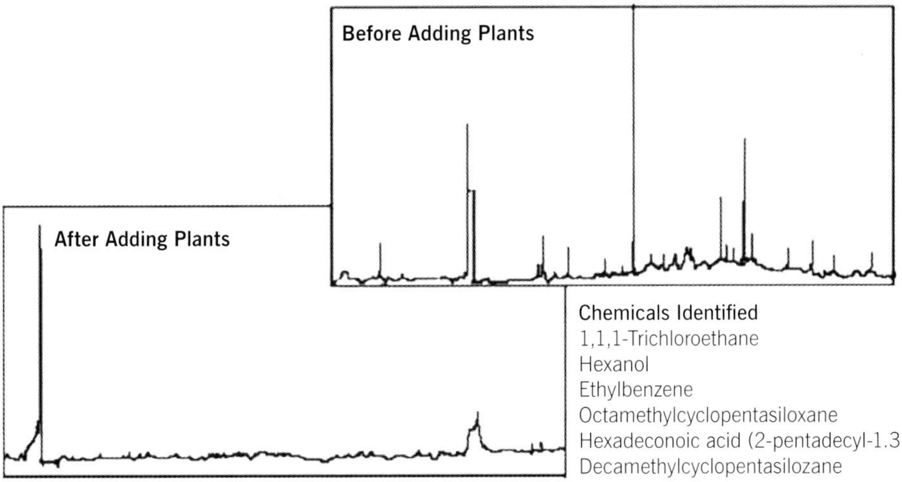

Chemicals Identified
1,1,1-Trichloroethane
Hexanol
Ethylbenzene
Octamethylcyclopentasiloxane
Hexadeconoic acid (2-pentadecyl-1.3 dio)
Decamethylcyclopentasilozane
Dodecamethylcyclohexasiloxane

Chemicals Identified
1,1-Dibromo-2-chloro-2-fluorocyclopropane

FIG. 2.6

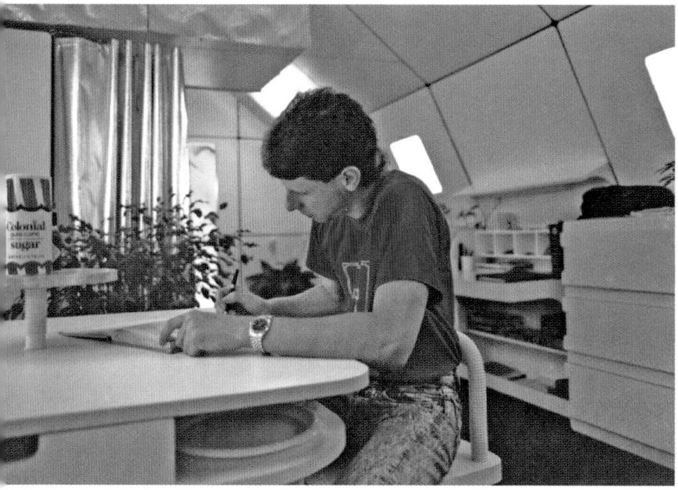

FIG. 2.7

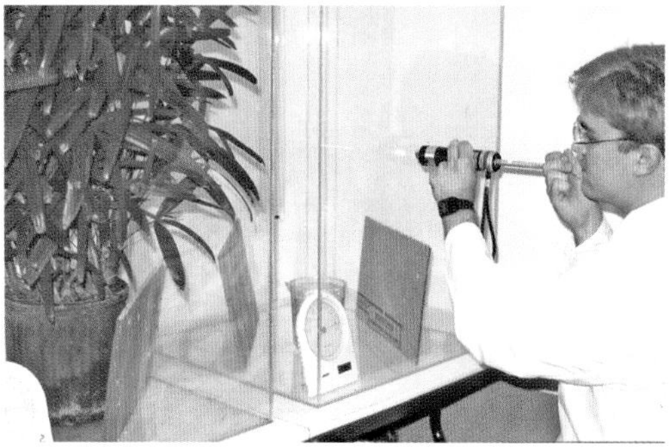

FIG. 2.8

constructed two Plexiglas test chambers. Scientists placed two sections of interior panelling comprising urea-formaldehyde resins into each chamber. A lady palm (*Rhapis excelsa*) was added to one chamber and the other chamber, serving as a control chamber, did not contain any plant. Plants, through their natural process of transpiration (emission of water vapour from leaves), cause humidity to rise in sealed chambers. To equalize humidity in both chambers, a beaker of water was placed in the plant-free chamber (Fig. 2.8).

As shown in Table 2.1, the lady palm removed formaldehyde that continuously off-gassed from the panelling sections. Temperature influenced the rate at which formaldehyde off-gassed from the panelling. The greater the temperature, the more rapidly formaldehyde was released. There was no removal of formaldehyde in the control chamber.

The lady palm showed no ill effects after extended exposure to formaldehyde. In fact, the lady palm increased its ability to remove formaldehyde as its exposure time increased. These studies indicated that plant root microbes had rapidly mutated and adapted to the presence of formaldehyde and had contributed significantly to the chemical removal process. Further studies sought to determine the extent of plant root and soil microbe involvement in the removal of chemicals. Formaldehyde and xylene were introduced individually into sealed chambers containing plants having either exposed soil or soil covered with sterilized sand. The studies showed that 50 to 65 per cent of VOC removal could be attributed to root and soil microbes. These findings indicate that both plants and the microbes around their

TABLE 2.1
ACCUMULATION OF FORMALDEHYDE INSIDE SEALED CHAMBERS CONTAINING PANELLING SECTIONS

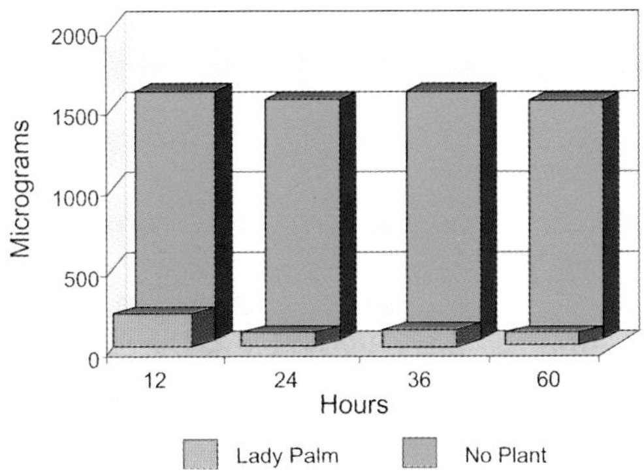

roots and in the soil contribute significantly to the removal of VOCs.

To further show the important role of soil microbes in reducing formaldehyde concentrations, researchers placed a dwarf azalea (*Rhododendron simsii 'Compacta'*) into a sealed chamber and tested its ability to remove formaldehyde. The azalea was then removed from its container and the container of soil was placed back into the chamber. Formaldehyde removal was reduced by 22 per cent after two days and 70 per cent after thirty days. Soil bacterial counts showed that without their host plant, the microbial population also decreased. The plant's root system is thus essential for providing an environment conducive for the growth of microbes. When plants are removed from the potting soil, the ability to remove formaldehyde from the air slowly decreases.

Due to the presence of microbes in the rhizosphere, interior plants are not damaged when exposed to high concentrations of VOCs but continue to improve in their ability to remove chemicals over time. The root/soil microbes rapidly adapt, producing new generations of microbes that are even more effective in using the chemicals as a source of food and energy. Scientists at the University of Technology in Sydney, Australia, later conducted similar studies and obtained similar results. The ability of soil microbes to degrade organic chemicals has been known for many years. Among the most effective microbes in degrading organic chemicals is *Pseudomonas* sp., commonly found around plant roots.

Studies show that both the plant leaves and root microbes contribute to the removal of VOCs from the indoor environment. It has been well-documented that plant leaves can absorb, metabolize and/or translocate certain VOCs to the root microbes where they are broken down. Studies show that 90 per cent of these substances are converted into sugars, new plant material and oxygen. Scientists at the GSF-National Research Center for Environment and Health in Neuherberg, Germany, produced the most definitive study yet on this phenomenon. They used radioactive carbon tracers to follow how the spider plant (*Chlorophytum comosum L.*) was able to break down and destroy formaldehyde.

The other mechanism plants employ to move air down to their root system is transpiration. While moving water up from their roots to their leaves, a small convection current is created pulling air down to the root zone. Through this process, a plant not only moves atmospheric gases such as oxygen and nitrogen to its root zone, but also the airborne chemicals. Because of this action, generally a plant with a high transpiration rate is more effective in its VOC removal capacity.

Hydroculture

In hydroponics, water and nutrients flow past the plant's roots intermittently and it is primarily used in commercial agricultural food production. Hydroculture, on the other hand, simply means 'water culture'. However, the two terms are often mistakenly interchanged. Hydroculture consists of a water-tight container, pebbles as a growth substrate and a constant water level in the container. Some hydroculture systems also use an inexpensive 'liner pot' that sits inside a decorative container (Fig. 2.9). The benefits are obvious in that the inner pot can simply be lifted out and placed in another decorative container. It also provides a simple means to rotate various plants without having to move the heavier outside container or to re-pot the plant.

The majority of indoor plants in European countries are grown in hydroculture. Other countries have been slower to accept this practice. It is thought to be too complicated or too scientific, when in reality it is a much simpler, cleaner concept. The determining factors in its lack of acceptance have been cost and availability. Most hydroculture systems currently sold in the US are imported from Europe. Manufacturing and shipping costs have made them cost-prohibitive to compete with soil-based planters. Growers have mistakenly believed that only expanded clay pebbles from Europe would function properly in a hydroculture system.

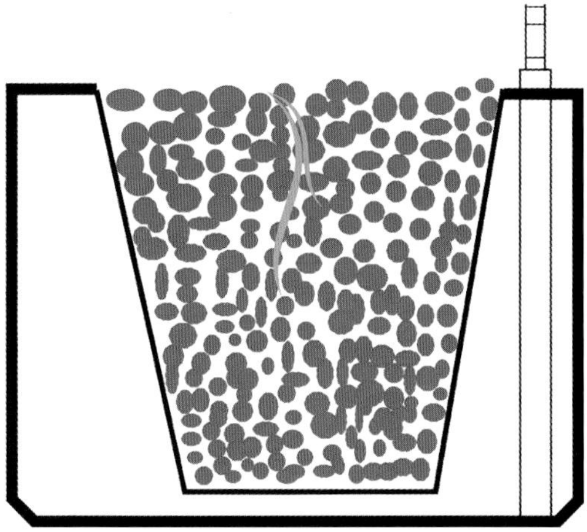

FIG. 2.9

Some of the many advantages of hydroculture are:

- Uses no soil. Inert pebbles are clean and odourless. Unlike soil, hydroculture does not harbour fungus spores that can become airborne in the ambient air. This is very helpful to allergy sufferers.
- Plants are not subject to soil-borne diseases or pests. The surface of soil-based plants is usually moist. As a result, they often harbour mould and the damp conditions encourage pests and disease.
- Water level indicator. Just keep the water level between the 'minimum' and 'maximum' markers. Because of the water reservoir, plants do not need caring for during weekends or vacations.
- Inert pebbles never need replacing. Unlike soil that needs refreshing or replacing, pebbles can be washed off and reused indefinitely. As such, pebbles are an environmentally sustainable product.
- Plants take up only the moisture they need. Because the pebbles provide a moist zone, plants having varying water requirements can be planted in the same container.
- Reduces the need to transplant. Nutrients and water are constantly available to the plant. Therefore, plants do not need to send out roots to search for them. So, they become less root-bound.
- Studies show that hydroculture plants are more effective in removing VOCs. For the process of transpiration, air can pass more easily down to the root zone through pebbles than through soil.

At this point, all previous interior plant studies were conducted using soil-based plants. So, WES set out to determine the viability of American expanded clay or shale products for use in hydroculture. Expanded clay and shale pebbles produced by Texas Industries, Inc. (TXI) headquartered in Dallas, Texas, were studied. Comparisons were made of the VOC removal rates of interior plants grown in potting soil and of those growing in hydroculture. Five common interior plants were chosen for the study (see Table 2.2).

TABLE 2.2

Common Name	Botanical Name
Areca Palm	*Dypsis lutescens*
Lady Palm	*Rhapis excelsa*
Rubber Plant	*Ficus robusta*
Peace Lily	*Spathiphyllum* sp.
Ficus alii	*Ficus binnendijkii 'Alii'*

FICUS ALII (*Ficus binnendijkii 'Alii'*)

Family: *Moraceae* (fig)
Origin: Thailand
Light: Medium light preferred
Temperature: Day: 16-24°C (60-75°F)
Night: 13-20°C (55-68°F)
Pests: Rarely, scale insects or mealybugs
Care: When using standard containers, water thoroughly then allow to dry before the next watering; drops yellow leaves when dry. In a sunroom or south-facing window, fertilize monthly. In darker settings, feed less often.

This ficus is rapidly becoming quite popular. Its slender dark green leaves make it an extremely attractive plant. It is much less finicky than the *Ficus benjamina*. There are three basic types: the bush (several stems from one pot), the standard tree (one trunk) and the braids (two or three entwined trunks).

When growing in soil, it is critical not to add too much water to this ficus. It is easier to maintain using sub-irrigation or hydroculture techniques. A magnificent large plant, its ability to help purify the air, ease of growth and resistance to insects make it an excellent choice for the home or office.

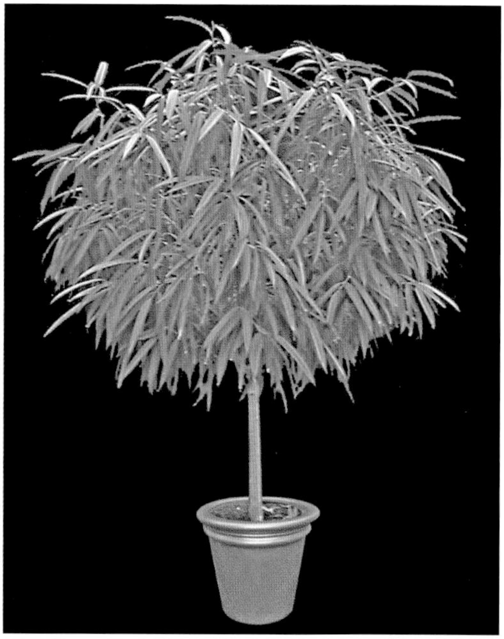

FIG. 2.10

TABLE 2.3
FORMALDEHYDE REMOVAL

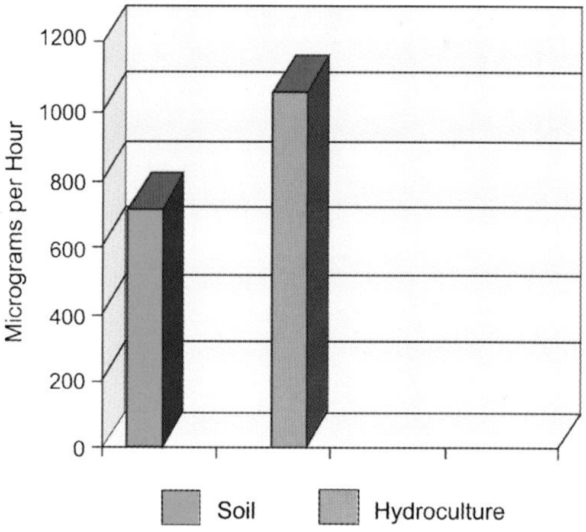

LADY PALM (*Rhapis excelsa*)

Family: *Arecaceae* (palm)
Origin: Southern China
Light: Tolerates low light
Temperature: 10-24°C (50-75°F)
Pests: Mostly pest-free but occasionally spider mites can create trouble.
Care: Water generously in spring and summer. In a warm, dry winter indoor environment, it may be necessary to water more frequently. Feed monthly with diluted liquid fertilizer.

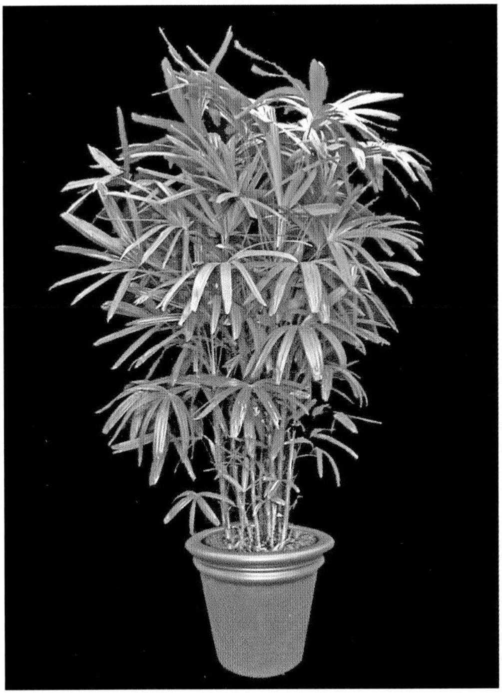

FIG. 2.11

The lady palm has fans that comprise between four and ten thick, shiny leaves. The leaves are connected to a brown, hairy main trunk by thin, arching stems. Lady palm is one of the easiest houseplants to care for and grows slowly. It is so popular in the United States that some commercial nurseries deal exclusively in its production.

When grown using sub-irrigation or hydroculture and tap water, some concentration of salt and minerals may accumulate in its leaf tips causing them to turn brown. The leaf tips can be trimmed with pinking shears (saw-toothed scissors) to remove the salt build-up and leave the tips with their natural green, serrated appearance.

TABLE 2.4
FORMALDEHYDE REMOVAL

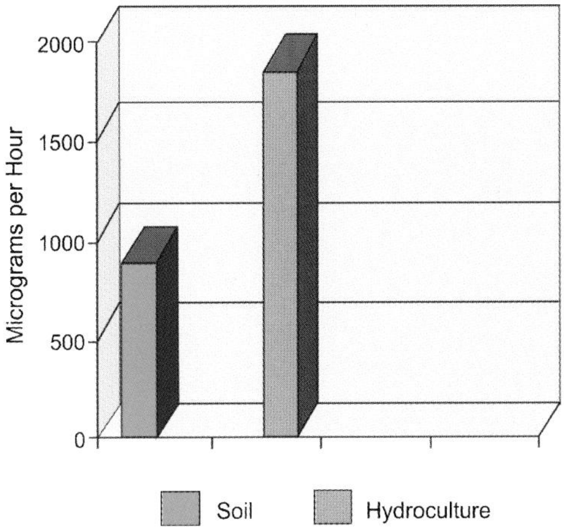

ARECA PALM (*Dypsis lutescens*)
*Formerly *Chrysalidocarpus lutescens*

Family: *Arecaceae* (palm)
Origin: Madagascar
Light: Semi-sun
Temperature: 18-24°C (65-75°F)
Pests: Spider mites and brown tips on fronds from over-dry atmosphere.
Care: Keep the root ball damp. Provide a complete fertilizer on a regular basis, except in winter. Mist regularly to give it a fresh appearance and to provide humidity to discourage insect infestation.

Also known as yellow palm or butterfly palm, the areca palm is one of the most popular and graceful palms. It is one of the faster-growing palms and features a cluster of cane-like stalks that produce feathery, yellow-green fronds.

The areca is consistently rated among the best houseplants for removing all indoor air toxins tested and has a high transpiration rate. A 6 ft (1.8 m) areca palm transpires approximately 1 quart (one litre) of water every twenty-four hours. As a result, it is more suited to hydroculture or sub-irrigation as these methods require less frequent watering. Its high ratings and popularity make the areca one of the top 'eco-friendly' houseplants.

TABLE 2.5
FORMALDEHYDE REMOVAL

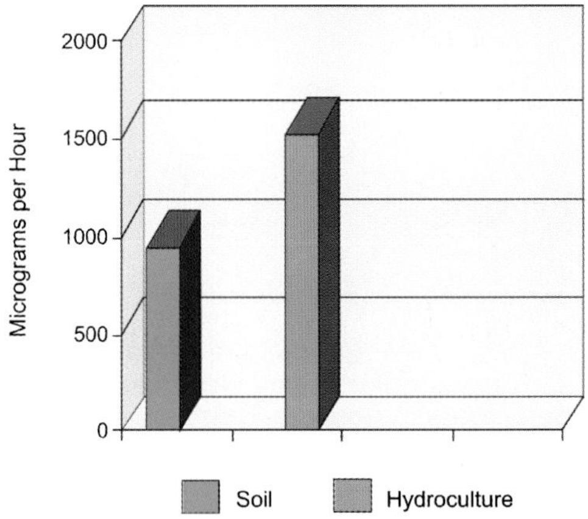

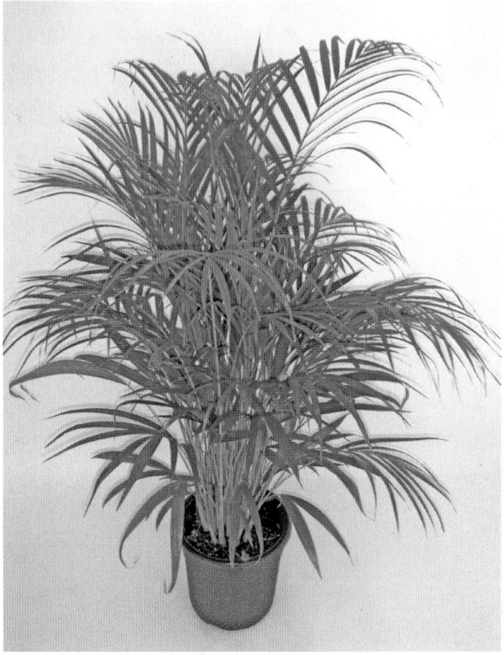

FIG. 2.12

RUBBER PLANT
(*Ficus robusta 'Burgundy'*)
*Formerly *Ficus elastica*

Family: *Moraceae* (fig)
Origin: India and Malaya
Light: Semi-sun to semi-shade
Temperature: 16-27°C (60-80°F); will tolerate temps as low as 5°C (40°F) for short periods.
Pests: Scale insects, mealybugs
Care: Feed regularly during the summer months only. Water regularly from mid-summer to fall, allowing the soil to dry slightly between two sessions of watering; then water sparingly. The rubber tree does not tolerate overwatering. It grows well in hydroculture.

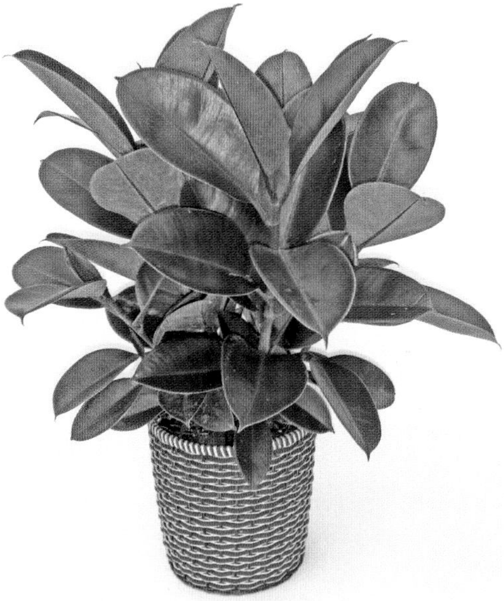

FIG. 2.13

The rubber plant's name is derived from its thick, dark-green leaves that contain rubber-like latex. It was a favourite plant of the Victorians and remains equally popular today. The rubber plant will survive in less light than most plants its size and will tolerate cool temperatures. It is an excellent plant for removing airborne chemical toxins from the indoor environment.

TABLE 2.6
FORMALDEHYDE REMOVAL

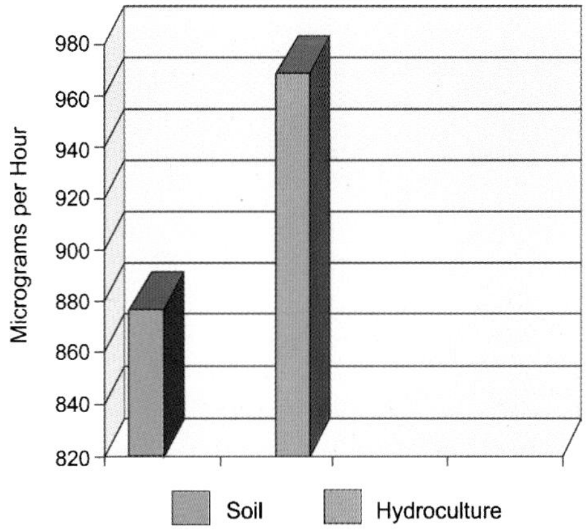

PEACE LILY (*Spathiphyllum* sp. *'Mauna Loa Supreme'*)

Family: *Araceae* (*Arum*)
Origin: Central America
Light: Semi-sun to semi-shade
Temperature: Day: 16-24°C (60-75°F); Night: 13-20°C (55-68°F)
Pests: If the air is too dry, it is susceptible to scale insects and spider mites; mealybugs.
Care: Feed regularly from spring to fall but less in winter. Wash the leaves occasionally to prevent insect attack. The peace lily performs exceptionally well in hydroculture or sub-irrigation.

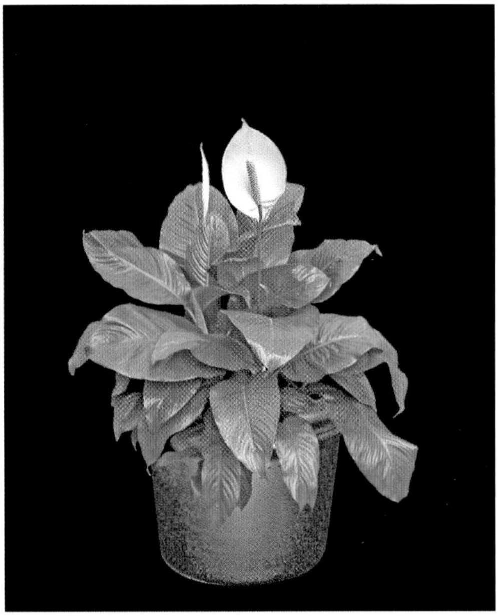

FIG. 2.14

The peace lily sends up stiff, erect stalks that produce white spathes. These spathes unfold to reveal the plant's true flower. The flower may be cut out to prevent the release of pollen and the spathe will continue unharmed for weeks. This plant, with its lush tropical foliage, is one of only a few plants that will reliably bloom indoors.

The peace lily excels in the removal of alcohols, acetone, trichloroethylene, benzene and formaldehyde. It has a high transpiration rate and needs watering less often in hydroculture. Because of its ability to remove indoor air pollutants and its all-round excellent qualities, the peace lily should always be included when seeking a variety of indoor plants.

TABLE 2.7
FORMALDEHYDE REMOVAL

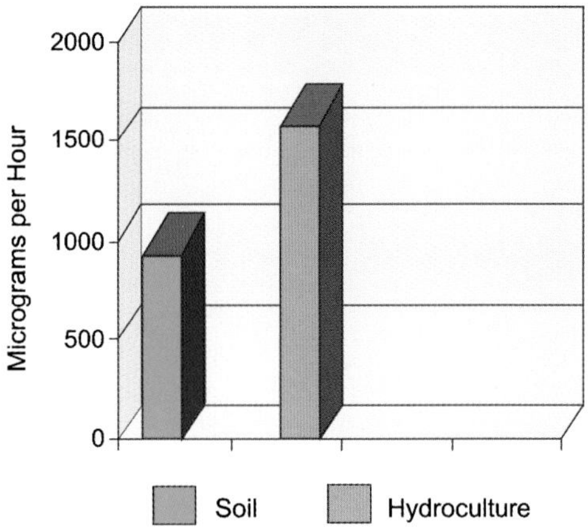

Tests conducted in an energy-efficient home sought to determine the influence of temperature and humidity on the transpiration rate (water loss) of plants. Studies using an areca palm (*Dypsis lutescens*) measuring 56 inches (142 cm) in height and growing in a 14 inch (36 cm) diameter hydroculture container was monitored for water loss at varying rates of humidity and temperature. As shown in Table 2.8, both factors affect transpiration rates. Generally, the relative humidity seemed to have the greater effect. The lower the humidity, the greater the water loss as the plant tried to raise humidity by emitting more water vapour. The indoor environment is notorious for having dangerously low relative humidity levels, especially during winter months when heating systems dry the air. Plants will add needed moisture to the air as they rapidly transpire in the low relative humidity of the indoor environment.

Studies were also conducted to determine whether high humidity levels inside plant chambers could contribute to formaldehyde removal. Comparative studies were conducted under identical conditions except that a desiccant was placed inside the plant chamber to reduce humidity. Insignificant differences were noted in the formaldehyde removal rates in both chambers. Therefore, it was concluded that humidity levels in the chambers played little or no role in formaldehyde removal.

Some sceptics expressed a concern that interior plants might increase the levels of mould spores and other airborne microbes. To address these concerns, portions of a tightly sealed, energy-efficient home located in South Mississippi served as 'real world' test chambers. A plant-filled sunroom and an adjacent living room served as test chambers in two separate studies, each three months

TABLE 2.8
TRANSPIRATION RATES OF A LARGE ARECA PALM GROWN IN HYDROCULTURE

Average Water Loss 24-Hour Period (oz)	(ml)	Average Relative Temperature (°F)	(°C)	Average Room Relative Humidity %
30.43	900	73	22.8	36.7
22.32	660	73	22.8	52.0
22.82	675	81	27.2	57.0
18.60	550	76	24.4	62.0

in duration and at different seasons of the year. A plant-free bedroom, located in another section of the home, served as a control.

Although humidity was higher in the plant-filled sunroom, airborne microbial counts were greater in the plant-free bedroom. In fact, they were an amazing 50 per cent greater in the bedroom. When placed in sufficient quantities, interior plants can influence airborne microbial populations in the indoor environment. Scientists have now conclusively shown that interior plants can 1) reduce VOCs, 2) reduce mould spores and other airborne microbes, and 3) increase humidity within energy-efficient structures.

In other plant studies, researchers at Washington State University (USA) studied the impact of interior plants on dust. Their studies measured particulate matter in a computer lab and a small office. Interior plants, when present, were located around the sides of the room for a one-week period. Particulate matter was measured in both rooms on various surfaces away from the plants. Dust accumulations were significantly less when plants were present. Dust was reduced by as much as 20 per cent when plants were placed in the rooms. This study confirmed that plants, when present in numbers commonly found indoors, can effectively reduce dust accumulations. Although the exact mechanisms plants employ to reduce dust accumulations are not known, scientists theorize that negative ions produced by plants may attract airborne particulate matter. Other studies are investigating this phenomenon further.

How Many Plants?

An often-asked question is how many plants are needed to maintain good indoor air quality? Unfortunately, there is not really a simple, definitive answer to this question. Air quality varies from building to building and may even vary from room to room. The amount of synthetic materials used in building materials and furnishings has great variances. Therefore, the amount of VOCs outgassing also fluctuates significantly. As we have learned, other factors such as temperature can greatly affect outgassing rates. The only means of determining exactly what chemicals are present in the indoor environment is through sophisticated analyses. The professionals and the scientific equipment needed to perform these tests often make the process cost-prohibitive. A simple rule is to just place as many plants as space, lighting, etc., will allow.

By using EPA datum derived from their monitoring of public access buildings for VOC levels and data obtained from VOC removal chamber studies, one can obtain a realistic estimate of the number of plants needed to improve indoor air quality. Based upon these criteria, two areca palms or lady palms should remove sufficient VOCs to significantly improve the indoor air quality in an 848 cubic ft (24 cubic m) room.

Professor Margaret Burchett, Dr Ron Wood and colleagues at the University of Technology, Sidney, Australia, are conducting extensive studies under 'real world' conditions in an effort to obtain a more accurate number of interior plants required to improve indoor air quality in a given area. Initial tests were conducted to monitor VOC levels in sixty offices, some of which contained a variety of interior plants and other offices had no plants present. Preliminary results showed a VOC reduction of 50 to 75 per cent in the offices where plants were present. These encouraging findings give further proof of the ability of interior plants to improve indoor air quality. The scientists are continuing this important research.

Plant-based Air Filters

In our modern, fast-paced society, plant-filled rooms help us keep in touch with nature. Just the ability to view living plants enhances our psychological and physiological well-being. However, in many buildings today, the amount of space allotted for the placement of plants is limited. But even this obstacle is surmountable.

Scientists at NASA's Stennis Space Center originally developed the concept of placing a plant in a mixture of soil and activated carbon and mechanically moving air down to the plant's roots. A working model equalled the VOC removal capacity of fifteen regularly grown interior plants (see Fig. 2.5).

In 1990, WES scientists set about to further develop this bio-technology. The first plant-based air filter did not use soil but a substrate consisting of expanded shale or clay, activated carbon and zeolite (see Fig. 2.15).

These soil-free filters employed a mechanical fan to pull air down through the highly adsorptive substrate in which an interior plant was grown. The substrate traps

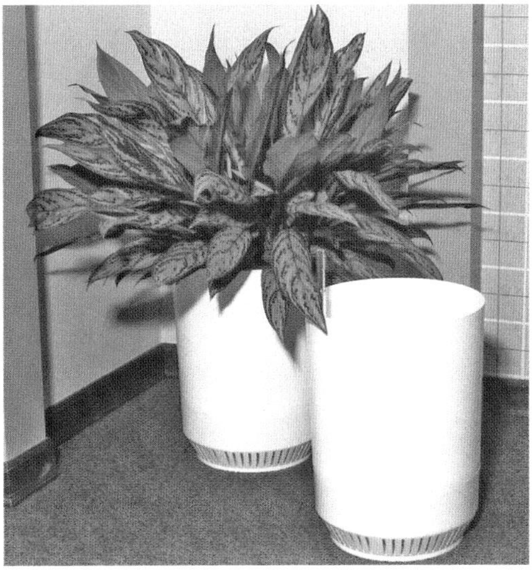

FIG. 2.15

any airborne contaminants, where the naturally occurring microbes biologically break down the trapped chemicals. The plant and microbes use these end products as a source of food and energy. In these filters, the plant's primary function is to serve as a host for the microbes. A bio-regenerative or self-cleaning filter is thus created since the microbes rapidly mutate and adapt to become more efficient with exposure. As a result, the filter media never becomes saturated or needs replacing, except under extreme conditions. The cleaned air is then returned to the room by the fan motor. This filter proved to be highly effective in removing formaldehyde and other VOCs from sealed test chambers and its efficiency increased as the microbes adapted to chemical exposure. A comparison of formaldehyde removal by a new filter and a two-year-old filter is shown in Table 2.9.

TABLE 2.9
REMOVAL OF FORMALDEHYDE BY PLANT/FAN AIR FILTER

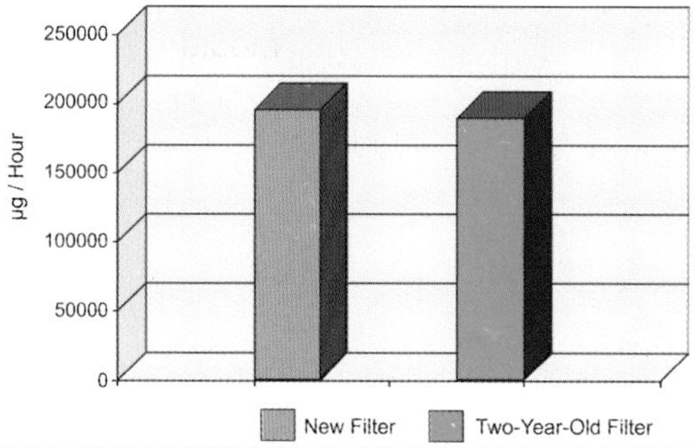

The first filter had several drawbacks. The fan motor was noisy and it was difficult to replace the plants. As a result, marketing of the filter was not successful.

WES later licensed the technology to Actree Corporation, a Japanese engineering and manufacturing company. Jointly, the two companies made further refinements. Actree Corporation now produces and markets in Japan a small, portable air filter termed the 'EcoPlanter' (see Figs. 2.16 and 2.17).

The EcoPlanter employs a quiet two-speed fan and contains an inner pot that can be easily removed for plant replacement. Also, as a final step in the EcoPlanter, filtered air passes a germicidal ultraviolet (UV) light

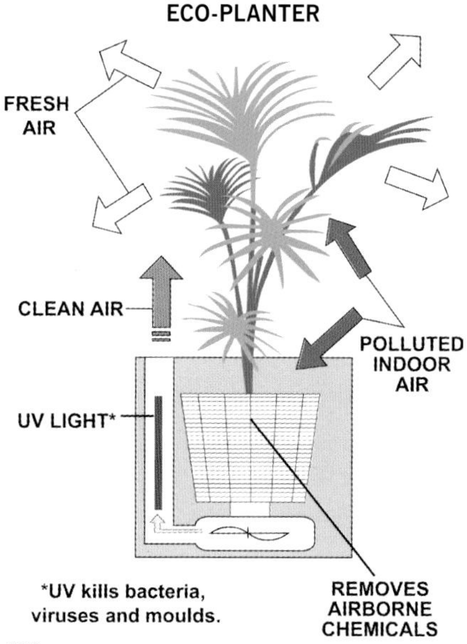

FIG. 2.16

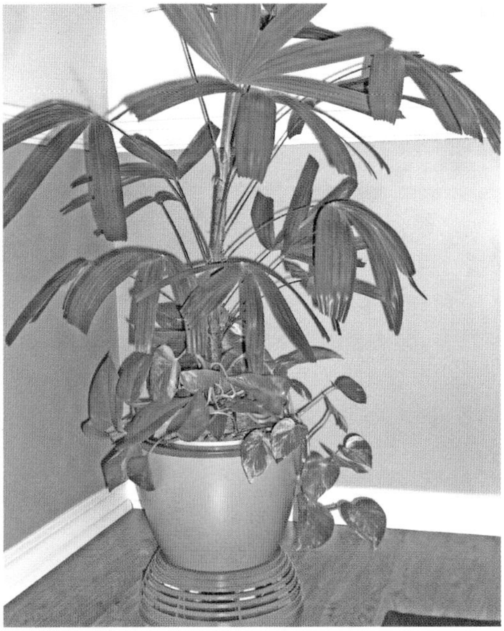

FIG. 2.17

TABLE 2.10
REMOVAL OF FORMALDEHYDE

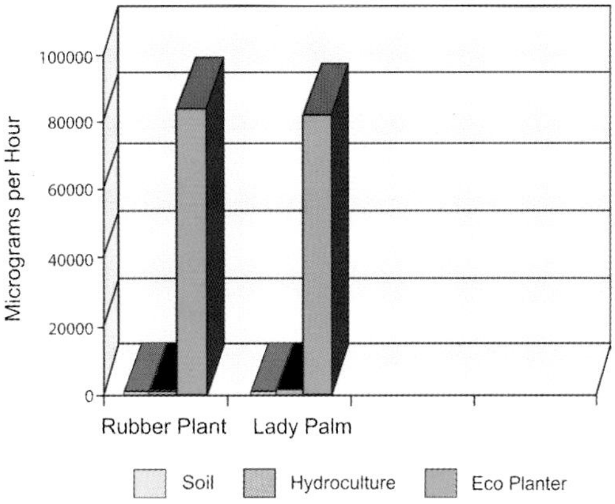

source to reduce or eliminate any remaining moulds, bacteria and viruses before the air is returned to the room. The EcoPlanter is an attractive planter/air filter that increases the VOC removal capacity of a single interior plant by as much as 100 times (see Table 2.10).

Most conventional air filtration devices in the market today use activated carbon and/or high-efficiency particulate arrester (HEPA) filters. These filters are limited only to trapping airborne pollutants and do nothing to destroy them. These filters become saturated and rely upon a strict maintenance routine to work properly. Often, due to neglect or high costs of replacement filters, proper maintenance is not done. If an activated carbon filter is not replaced before becoming saturated, toxic chemicals trapped on its surface may render the filter ineffective. Even worse, the chemicals may be released back into the room; thus, creating an even greater airborne chemical concentration in the indoor environment.

If HEPA filters are not regularly replaced, they can become clogged and ineffective as a filtration device. Also, mould and other microbes trapped on the filter surface may flourish and multiply causing a potential health hazard. Pollutant-laden filters are often not disposed of in an environmentally friendly manner. EcoPlanters, having no filters to replace, overcome these problems. Unfortunately, due to manufacturing and shipping costs, the EcoPlanter was never introduced into markets other than Japan.

As discussed in the previous chapter, temporary housing was provided by FEMA to thousands of victims of Hurricanes Katrina and Rita along the Gulf Coast. Due to the bad air quality within the trailers, the residents often sought medical help for a variety of ailments such as respiratory problems, asthma, rashes, dizziness, etc. After conducting air quality tests, the Sierra Club determined that formaldehyde levels were excessively high due to the extensive use of particle board in the construction process. The World Health Organization (WHO) currently sets a safe range of formaldehyde indoors at 0.05 parts per million (ppm) or less.

In October 2006, WES and the local Sierra Club headed by Becky Gillette placed an EcoPlanter inside a FEMA trailer located in Bay St Louis, Mississippi. The trailer was the temporary home of a young couple and their small child. Samples taken before placement of the EcoPlanter showed a formaldehyde concentration of 0.18 ppm. Within several days, tests revealed that the EcoPlanter had reduced the formaldehyde concentration to 0.03 ppm. All samples were collected by the residents and shipped to an independent laboratory for analyses. These preliminary findings revealed the potential for plant-based air filters to remove harmful formaldehyde within an indoor environment.

In an effort to make the plant-based air filter technology more economically viable, WES is currently designing an enhanced version that offers a larger filter to provide even greater filtering capacity as well as allow for larger plants or multiple plants to grow within the filter.

Whole Building Concept

Without question, the ultimate goal has always been to further plant-based air filter technology whereby the air is treated for the whole building. Any small, portable filter has a limited range of effectiveness. As a result, further studies have led to the development of a 'whole building' concept using modular planter systems.

Modular planter systems are much larger in scale, allow for automatic watering and provide space for a greater diversity of plants. Most importantly, they may be connected to the building's HVAC system so that during the internal air-exchange process, the air recycles through various planter modules, stripping the air of pollutants, before returning to the indoor environment. This process reduces the need for outside ventilation that carries its own pollutants into the indoor environment and has other inherent problems.

There are two types of modular planters: passive modular planters and forced-air modular planters. A passive modular planter system located in a sunroom has functioned successfully in Dr Wolverton's home since 1989. Through the years, analyses show undetectable VOC levels and a 50 per cent reduction in airborne moulds and bacteria (Figs. 2.18 and 2.19).

Forced-air modular planters make use of a fan motor to move air more rapidly through the planters, providing increased filtration capacity. These modular planters may also pass the air by an ultraviolet (UV) light to destroy any remaining moulds and bacteria in the air. Because these filters clean airborne contaminants more rapidly, fewer plants are needed. Conceptual drawings are shown of forced-air modular planters that will provide air filtration for entire rooms and whole buildings (Figs. 2.20 and 2.21).

The goal is to place modular planters – some passive modular planters and others having forced air filtration – throughout large

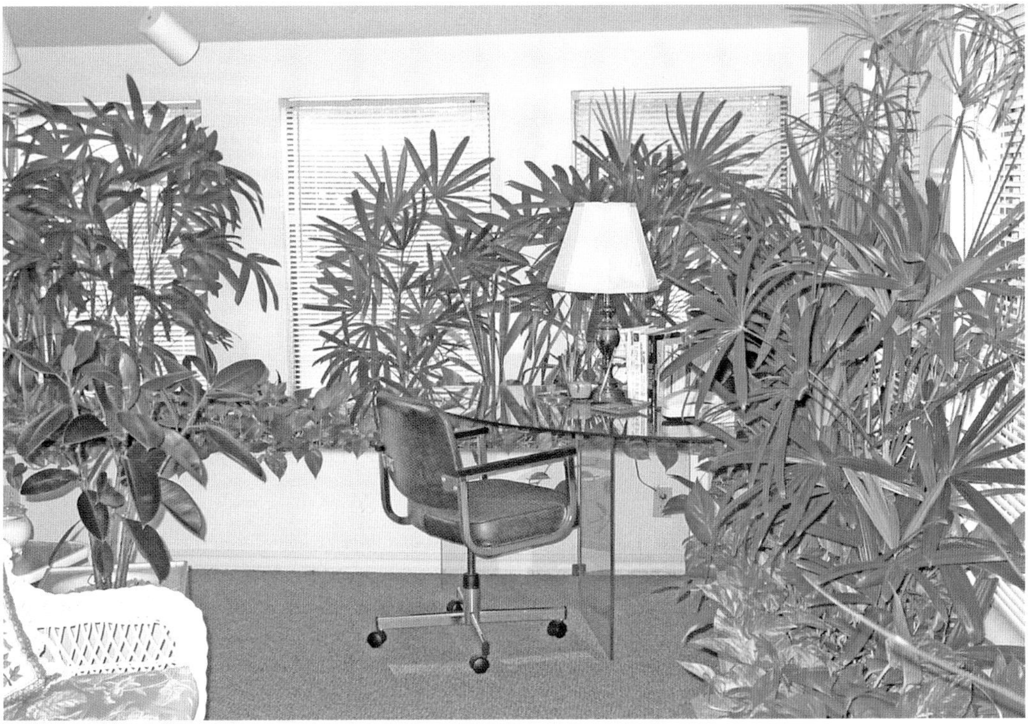

FIG. 2.18

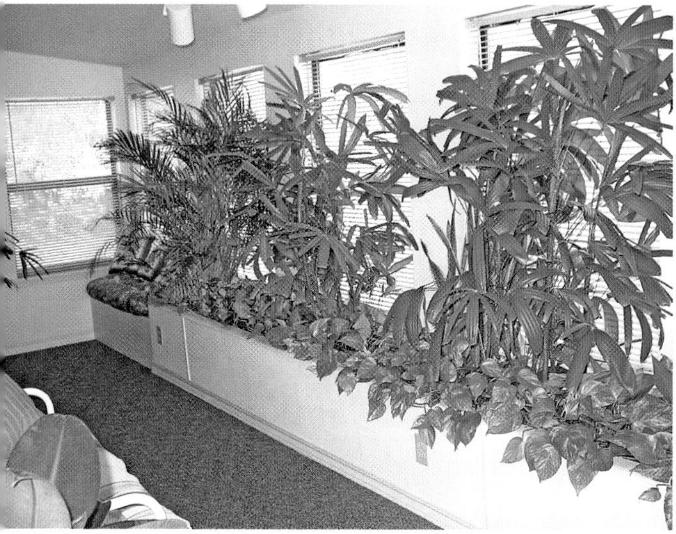
FIG. 2.19

buildings near windows, in atriums or in rooftop greenhouses. While an attractive addition to interior spaces, the filters will quietly filter the air of harmful pollutants before it is returned into a room or building. Interior-scape industry professionals, who already place and maintain plants in buildings, will be able to attend to the plants during their regular plant maintenance schedules.

As these filters allow for greater recycling of air and reduced ventilation, an exciting aspect of the technology is energy savings.

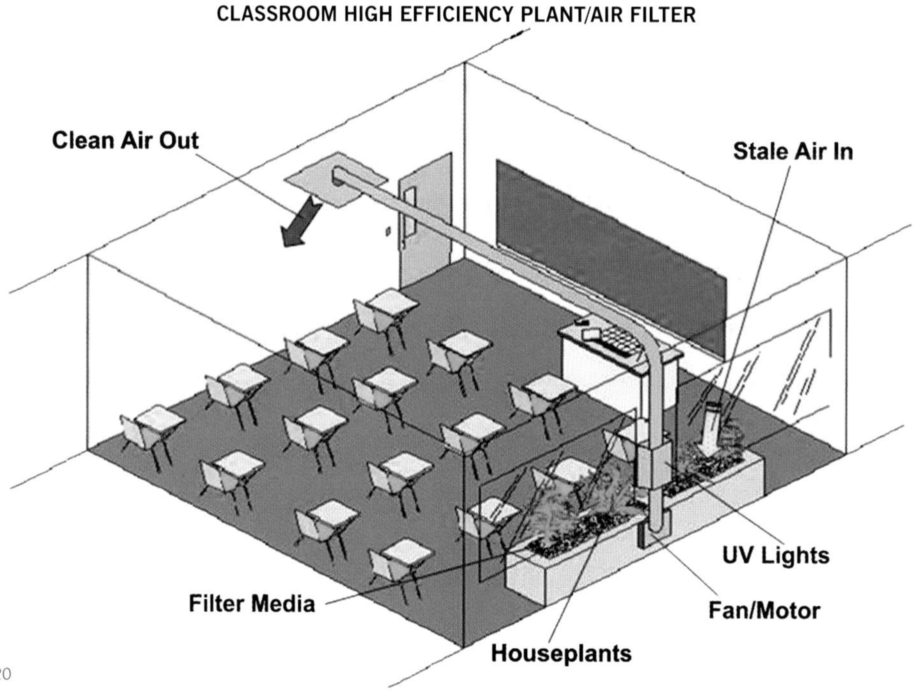

FIG. 2.20

With today's spiralling energy costs, reducing energy consumption within a building is vital. However, the most important function is to help alleviate the build-up of chemicals and other pollutants within the building that adversely affect its inhabitants.

Others have developed their own unique systems. One system is known by a variety of names, including green walls, living walls, bio walls or vertical gardens (see Figs. 2.22 and 2.23). These systems make use of the vertical space within a building and are attached to existing walls. Of these, some incorporate fans to draw the impure air

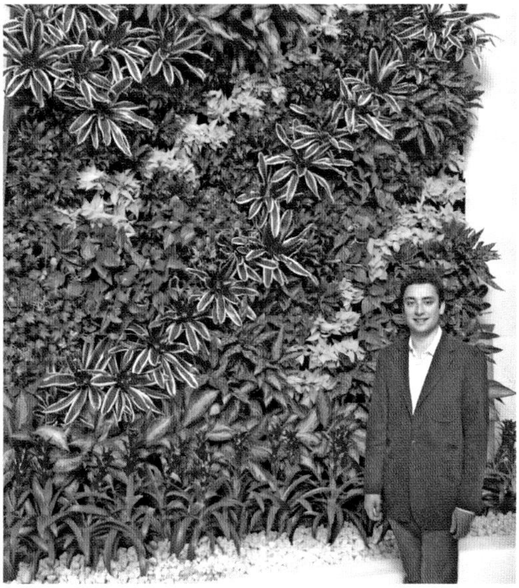

FIG. 2.22

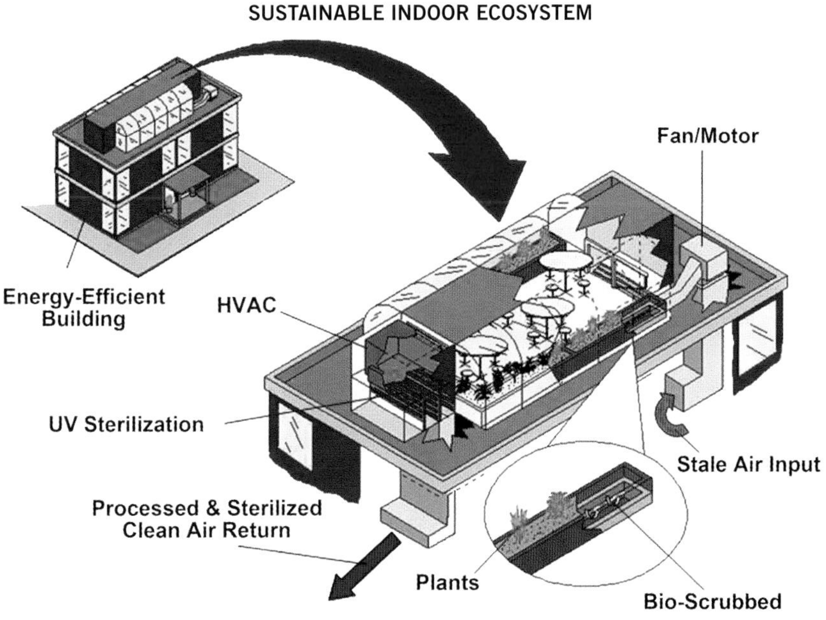

FIG. 2.21

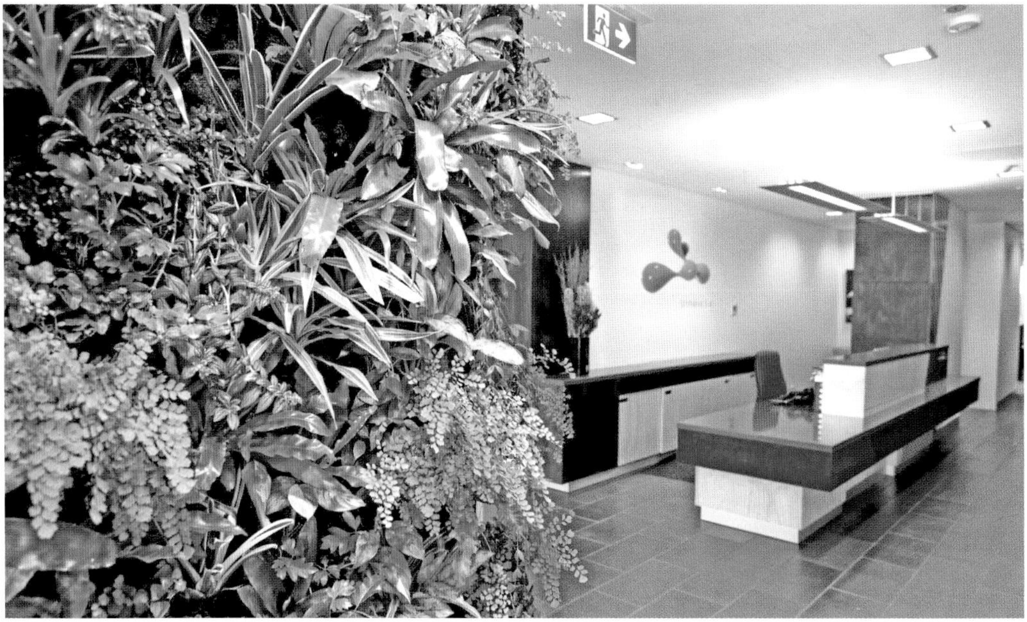

FIG. 2.23

through the wall and then circulate the clean air throughout the building, or only in a portion of the building, while others are inactive or passive walls and have no mechanized air circulation. These systems are gaining in popularity, especially in European countries.

All these biological systems depend upon microbes that naturally exist in the plants root systems to break down chemical pollutants. When coupled with the aesthetical and health-related benefits of placing plants within buildings, the future for plants and forced-air plant filters within the indoor environment is bright.

Continuing Education

In the late 1980s, PLANET, formerly known as ALCA, was the first to support more research into the use of plants to improve indoor environment. The industry continues to support education through the non-profit organization, Green Plants for Green Buildings (formerly, Plants at Work). The group is spearheading a national education campaign designed to educate professionals and the public about the benefits of interior plants in the workplace. One of the group's slogans nudges the building industry to include plants in their 'green building' designs: 'The building isn't green until the plants arrive!' The group is working closely with the American Institute of Architects (AIA), the National Association of Building Owners and Managers (BOMA) and the US Green Building Council (USGBC) to provide continuing education to building industry professionals. Their website is located at www.greenplantsforgreenbuildings.org.

The Plants for People organization, with offices in the United Kingdom, Germany and the Netherlands, has a similar objective. This group seeks to spread the knowledge of the benefits of plants in a work environment by supporting international research projects, collecting and publicizing relevant study results and communicating these results at symposiums and workshops. Their website is located at www.plants-for-people.org.

Green Buildings

The USGBC is a coalition of building industry leaders working to promote buildings that are environmentally responsible, energy efficient and healthy places in which to live and work. The standards set by the Leadership in Energy and Environmental Design (LEED) Green Building Rating System should be commended. Yet, living plants are not currently included in the certification standard. One would think that the 'green building' concept would try to closely mimic the existing 'green earth' where living plants purify and revitalize the earth's atmosphere. Green Plants for Green Buildings has received official approval from the USGBC for its curriculum on the benefits of plants for green building professionals. As the LEED programme evolves, it is hoped that consideration will be given to the benefits that live plants offer to human health and well-being in built spaces. Then and only then will buildings be truly green.

Going Green in the United States

Construction of the Bank of America Tower in New York City is touted as the world's greenest skyscraper. Scheduled for completion in 2009, the building's designers expect it to be the largest structure to earn the top-level 'platinum' rating from the USGBC. While the building is to incorporate many of the latest technologies in energy-use reduction and water conservation, the only mention of any living plants is a one-acre green roof (outside the building). The air filtration system is designed to filter suspended particulate matter and VOCs from the outside air before it is circulated throughout the building and then filtered again before release into the outside environment.

Outside air is to be filtered through MERV-15 rated air filters to remove particulate matter as small as 2.5 microns in diameter. According to Scott Frank, a partner with Jaros Baum & Bolles – the mechanical engineers

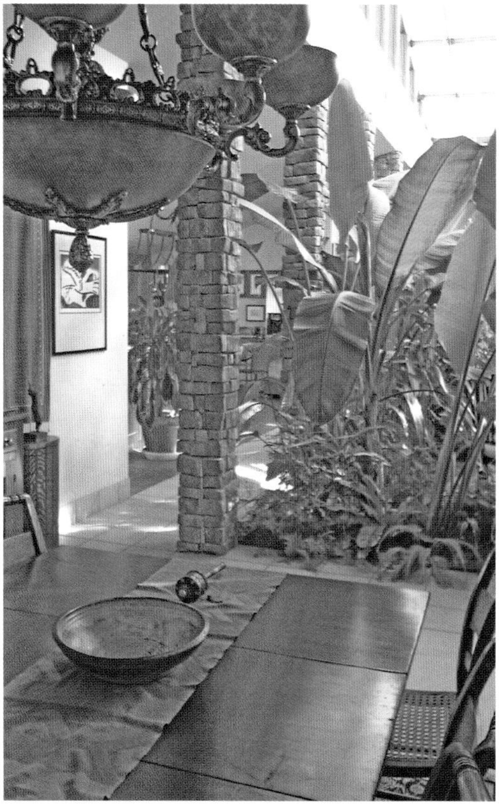

FIG. 2.24

on the project – a second filter, an activated carbon filter, will remove VOCs. However, there does not appear to be any bio-regenerative process that would reduce ventilation rates by purifying, revitalizing and recycling air internally. The costs associated with heating and cooling the filtered outside air could be significant. Also, regularly replacing activated carbon and particulate filters can impact building maintenance costs.

Going Green in India

The Paharpur Business Centre and Software Technology Incubator Park consists of a 50,000 sq ft (4,647 sq m) building complex located in Nehru Place Greens, a premier commercial centre in New Delhi, India. This complex houses many Fortune 500 companies that have established operations in India (www.pbcnet.com).

The outside air in New Delhi is heavily polluted, yet the air inside this complex is pure and fresh. This oasis is possible through the use of standard filtration devices such as air scrubbers, activated carbon filters, HEPA filters and dehumidifiers. Where this building differs from other energy-efficient buildings is that the filtered air passes through a greenhouse (home to more than 1,600 interior plants), for a second round of filtration, before its re-introduction into the office complex. The plants perform several functions: 1) Refresh the air by adding oxygen and negative ions; 2) Remove carbon dioxide exhaled by building occupants during respiration; and 3) Remove any remaining VOCs from the air. The company even has its own indoor air quality lab where the IAQ is continuously monitored for oxygen levels, humidity, etc. Suspended particulate matter and carbon dioxide readings both inside and outside the building are measured daily and the results posted on the company website.

As another tool in its efforts to provide pure, fresh air, the company purchased a six-acre tract adjacent to the complex. More than 2,000 trees were planted and the area converted into a beautiful park. This effort improved the ambient air quality by creating a lush micro-climate in the area. The complex and adjacent park has truly become a green 'oasis' within a concrete jungle. This unique IAQ programme is based on the pioneering research conducted by NASA at the John C Stennis Space Center in Mississippi during the 1980s.

CEO Kamal Meattle states that the company is now constructing the world's most energy-efficient building near New Delhi. The 1.7 million sq ft (157,992 sq m) commercial building will be complete with a 48,000 sq ft (4,461 sq m) duty-free shopping area and a fifty-room hotel. The building is to be a USGBC LEED Certified 'Platinum Green Building'. The plans call for the use of approximately 60,000 interior plants that will be placed throughout the building complex as well as in rooftop greenhouses containing both passive and forced-air filtration modular planters. The interior plants will primarily consist of areca palms (*Dypsis lutescens*) and snake plants (*Sansevieria* sp.). This building is scheduled for completion in 2011 and will be the largest energy-efficient building in the world to use interior plants as a major component of the air purification process (www.greenspaces.in).

In Agra, India, home to the Taj Mahal, a new 150-room Ramada Hotel is currently in the design phase. According to architect Joseph Kiriaty, this hotel will make use of modular planter systems located within the atrium and around the balconies to help provide clean, fresh air throughout the building. India is quickly becoming a world leader in the green building industry.

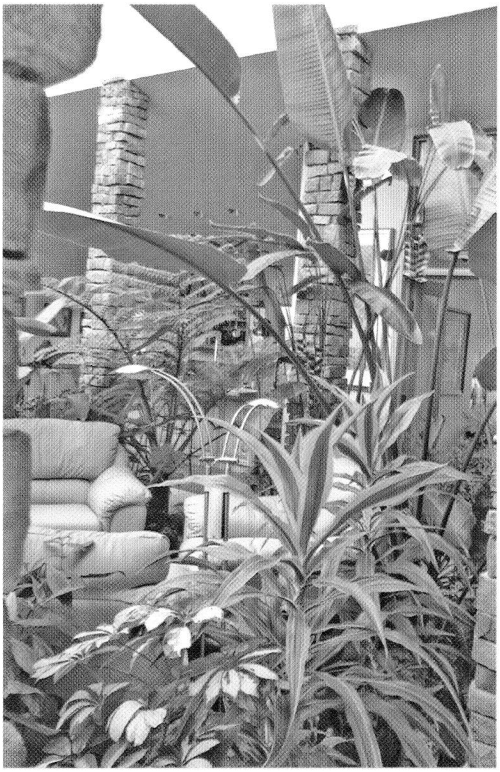

FIG. 2.25

Innovative Architects

Slowly but ardently, architects and the building industry are inching their way toward a more holistic approach to our living spaces. Cold, stark designs are losing favour as the 'closeness to nature' approach is now in vogue. Two architects who are at the forefront of bringing us closer to nature in our homes are Stuart Rose, Ph.D and Mason Edmunds. Their designs are just examples of many of the more progressive architects who are offering exciting new designs.

Dr Stuart Rose has built a unique cluster of 'Garden Atrium' homes, the first of which is located in Poquoson, Virginia. His designs have created one of the foremost energy-efficient and eco-friendly residential communities in the United States. By incorporating state-of-the-art technologies and a stunning indoor garden atrium, Dr Rose has made this Garden Atrium community truly 'green'. For more information, visit www.gardenatriums.com (see Figs. 2.24, 2.25 and 2.26).

Architect Mason Edmunds of Edmunds International has long incorporated the extensive use of interior plantings in his designs. As a behavioural architect, he places plants within built spaces with an equal emphasis on the physical and emotional benefits they provide to the residents. As an example, a private residence built in 1993

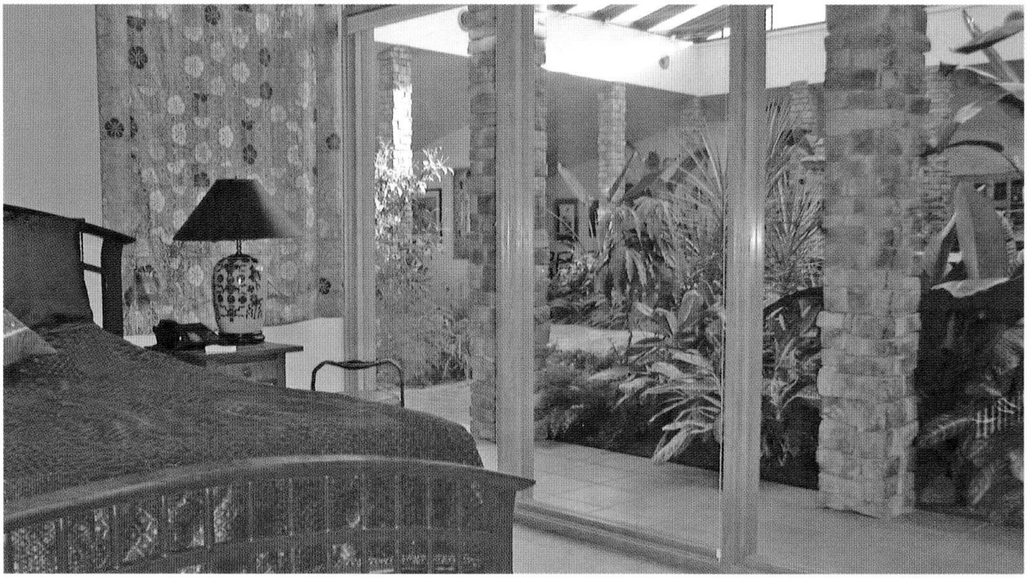

FIG. 2.26

utilizes over 1,150 tropical foliage plants as well as exotic plants to create a beautiful and serene environment. The lush plantings throughout the home provide emotional well-being while silently purifying the air within the home. For more information, visit www.edmundsintl.com (see Fig. 2.27).

SUMMARY

For centuries man has studied the complex biological processes taking place within a single, living plant. Even today, there is much to learn about the interaction between humans and plants. Exciting revelations in the last few decades have helped us realize that an interior plant, valued for its aesthetic beauty, quietly but efficiently works in the background to enhance our well-being. Scientists in Australia, Europe, Canada, India, China, South Korea and Japan continue to enhance the pioneering work of NASA and Dr B.C. Wolverton. Scientists have made many discoveries helping us understand the complexities of plants and how they can purify both air and water.

As we live in increasingly complex societies and living spaces, enveloped by synthetic materials and furnishings, it is even more vital to remain in contact with nature. The air we breathe today comprises many synthetic chemicals that were developed only a few decades ago. We are just beginning to understand the dangers these chemicals pose to our health. No one proposes that we abandon our modern lifestyle. However, we should seek to improve the quality of the air we breathe by bringing living plants indoors. By designing living plant systems into our modern buildings, we have the potential to not only produce healthy indoor air, but to also save on energy costs, increase worker productivity and reduce healthcare costs. Innovative high-efficiency plant filters are just one example of how, through man's ingenuity, we can harness the power of nature to enhance our lives and produce truly green buildings.

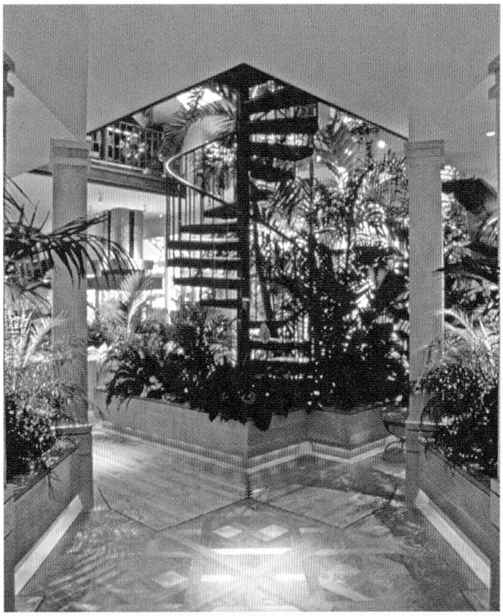

FIG. 2.27

Interior Plants for Human Health and Well-being

The cultivated garden has its basis rooted in man's desire to surround oneself with plants. In fact, the Persian word for garden is *paradise*, inferring that a garden is a source of pleasure. Gardens have two basic functions: a utilitarian function to meet human needs and an aesthetic one to be a place of beauty for relaxation and pleasure.

European and Asian societies have recognized for centuries that living in close proximity to plants and gardens is advantageous to human health. The practice of placing plants into containers originated in Greece and was a generally accepted practice towards the end of the fourth century BC. However, written documents show that the Egyptians began bringing plants indoors in the third century BC. The plants were placed in clay vessels and resided in inner courts for ornamental purposes.

In 1865, renowned American landscape architect Frederick Law Olmstead stated that an environment containing vegetation or other nature 'employs the mind without fatigue and yet exercises it; tranquilizes it and yet enlivens it; and thus, through the influence of the mind over the body, gives the effect of refreshing rest and reinvigoration to the whole system'. While throughout history many have recognized the positive effects of psychological and physiological well-being through human interaction with plants, few empirical studies had actually taken place.

Healthcare Facilities

Physicians in ancient Egypt prescribed walks in gardens for the mentally disturbed. During the Middle Ages, elaborate gardens were often created to help comfort the sick. In the nineteenth century, hospitals in Europe and America commonly displayed plants and provided garden settings for both patients and visitors. In fact, Dr Benjamin Rush, a signatory of the Declaration of Independence and considered to be the 'Father of American Psychiatry', reported that garden settings held curative effects for people with mental illness.

In more recent times, healthcare facilities seeking to house modern medical equipment, accommodate increased patient loads and reduce infection risk squeezed plants and gardens out of their buildings. As a result, most healthcare facilities became cold, impersonal institutions. They provided little in the way of creating a less stressful environment and offered even less to making the environment more conducive to healing or working.

Today, however, the growing practice of integrated medicine, where the mind-body connection is more respected, has stirred a renewed interest in returning plants and gardens to healthcare facilities to aid in the healing process. Dr Andrew Weil, a leading practitioner of integrative medicine states, 'one of the most important features of integrative medicine is its reconnection to nature as a source of healing'.

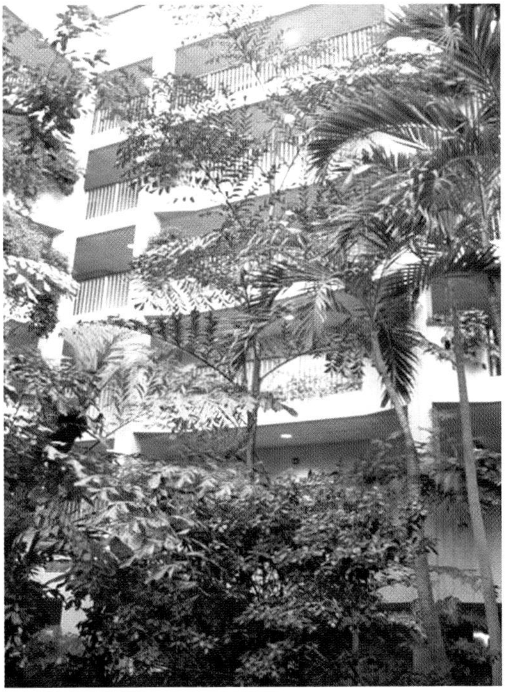

FIG. 3.1

Many hospitals, retirement homes, acute and chronic care inpatient centres and outpatient facilities now include the use of 'restorative gardens'. These gardens can range in scale from a collection of indoor plants in containers to roof gardens and even outdoor landscape. Many also incorporate the soothing effect of moving water whether in a small fountain or a constructed or natural stream.

One of the world's largest residential indoor rainforests is a 287-unit senior citizen residence called The Park at Vernon Hills, located in a North Chicago, Illinois suburb. The rainforest is larger than a football field (1.04 acres/0.42 hectares) and seven stories high (Fig. 3.1). It contains more than 7,000 trees and plants. It has walls blooming with passion fruit flowers, bleeding heart vines, and bougainvillea and chestnut vines. This rainforest creates a healthy living environment for residents by providing clean air and lush green foliage.

Dr Tomer Anbar, who conceived the therapeutic rainforest project, cites the air-purifying properties of interior plants when explaining the reason behind its creation. The facility opened in April 2000 and uses a five-million BTU heating and cooling system to help maintain a comfortable environment for residents and plants alike. A computer-controlled, 58,000 watt supplemental lighting system provides optimum lighting for the rainforest's major tree specimens. Many of the residents have stated that they believe the rainforest provides health benefits such as a decrease in respiratory problems and an improvement in sinus conditions and dry eyes (Fig. 3.2). Plants and overall landscape architectural design help to create an aesthetically pleasing, home-like, non-institutional setting as opposed to a medical or institutional setting.

Health Central, a hospital located in Ocoee, Florida, serves the greater Orlando area. It is unique both in its architecture and interior atrium. The six-storey main lobby atrium is planted with large palms and ficuses growing in a combination of structural and free-standing planters. Even more palms are planted in the lower-level food court and are visible from the atrium lobby. A fountain surrounded by bromeliads and ferns adds an abundance of refreshing negative air ions as well as a visual and acoustic feature. Nestled in the shade of the tall multi-headed palms is a grand piano from which can be heard soothing live music throughout the day. This is definitely much more calming and reassuring (Fig. 3.3) than the usual cold, impersonal hospital setting.

The Brent House located in New Orleans, Louisiana offers lodging to the general public with an emphasis on serving the needs of Ochsner Clinic Foundation's patients and their families. An enclosed six-storey atrium features fountains, lush tropical foliage,

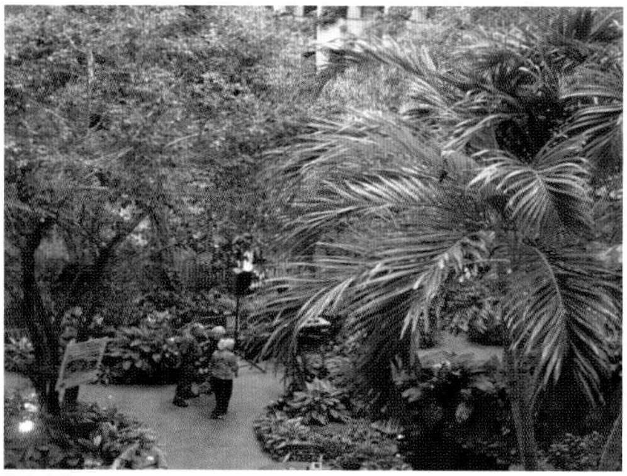

FIG. 3.2

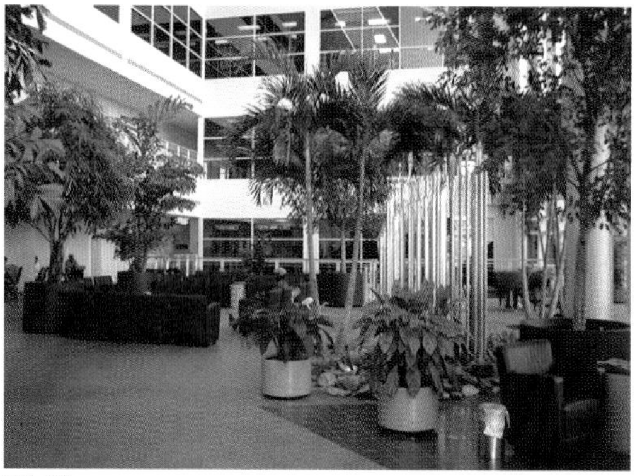

FIG. 3.3

gazebos and comfortable furnishings characteristic of both New Orleans and Latin American architecture. Located adjacent to all services offered by Ochsner, the Brent House provides a lush indoor garden that is available to both the clinic and the hospital. It offers a quiet, serene setting and promotes restorative healing and reflection (Fig. 3.4).

Takenaka Garden Afforestation, Inc., Tokyo's largest interior plant-scape company, has studied the research results regarding plants and their ability to improve indoor air quality. Kozaburo and Katsuko Takenaka, in conjunction with Dr Wolverton, have developed 'Ecology Gardens' for use in public buildings. Ecology gardens are indoor gardens that use a specially formulated growth media containing in part a mixture of activated charcoal and limestone. Studies show that plants in ecology gardens are more effective in the removal of VOCs than indoor gardens in regular, commercially produced potting soil. Ecology gardens are shown at two Tokyo hospitals: Jyuntendo Hospital (Fig. 3.5) and Showa University Hospital (Figs. 3.6 and 3.7).

Many healthcare facilities are now seeking to provide a more holistic approach to their medical practices, one that attends to the entire gamut of their patients' physical, mental and spiritual needs. Providing well-landscaped exteriors and lush interior gardens are major components in making this goal a reality. Besides being an optimal environment for healing, they offer workers a less stressful workplace.

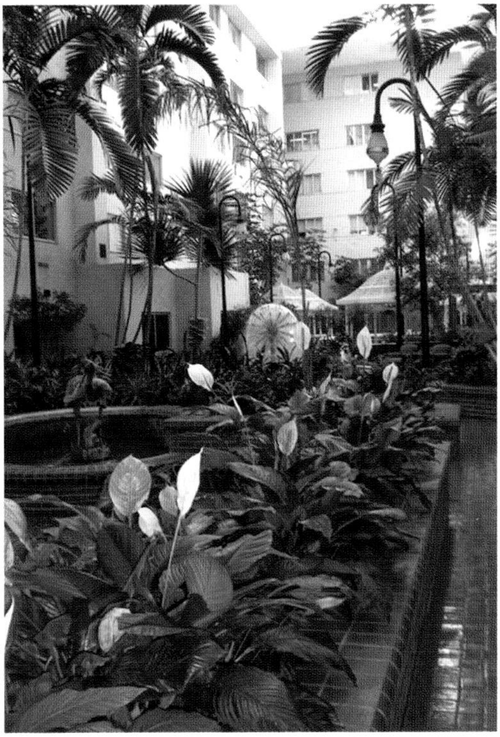

FIG. 3.4

Hospitality Industry

For many years plants have been placed in hotels, restaurants, offices and homes for their ambience. However, scientists in the US, Japan and several European countries have proven during recent years that plants play a far more significant role in our lives than just aesthetics.

The hospitality industry recognizes that providing a comfortable, soothing atmosphere is important for their guests. If guests are going to return for repeated stays, it is imperative that they leave relaxed and rejuvenated. One of the easiest ways to provide guests with a tranquil and inviting atmosphere is to surround them with living plants. In addition to a calming effect, studies show that plants also help minimize noise within interior spaces. In a study conducted by scientists at South Bank University in London, plants were shown to absorb background noise in buildings, resulting in a more comfortable environment for its occupants.

One of the most impressive displays of plants in a hotel setting is at the Opryland Hotel in Nashville, Tennessee (USA). The hotel features two large six-storey, semi-tropical indoor gardens covering 3.46 acres (1.4 hectares), with footpaths and walkways that allow guests to stroll past fountains, waterfalls and 50,000 tropical plants, including rare and exotic species (Fig. 3.8).

Rooms overlooking Opryland's interior gardens are always the first to be reserved by

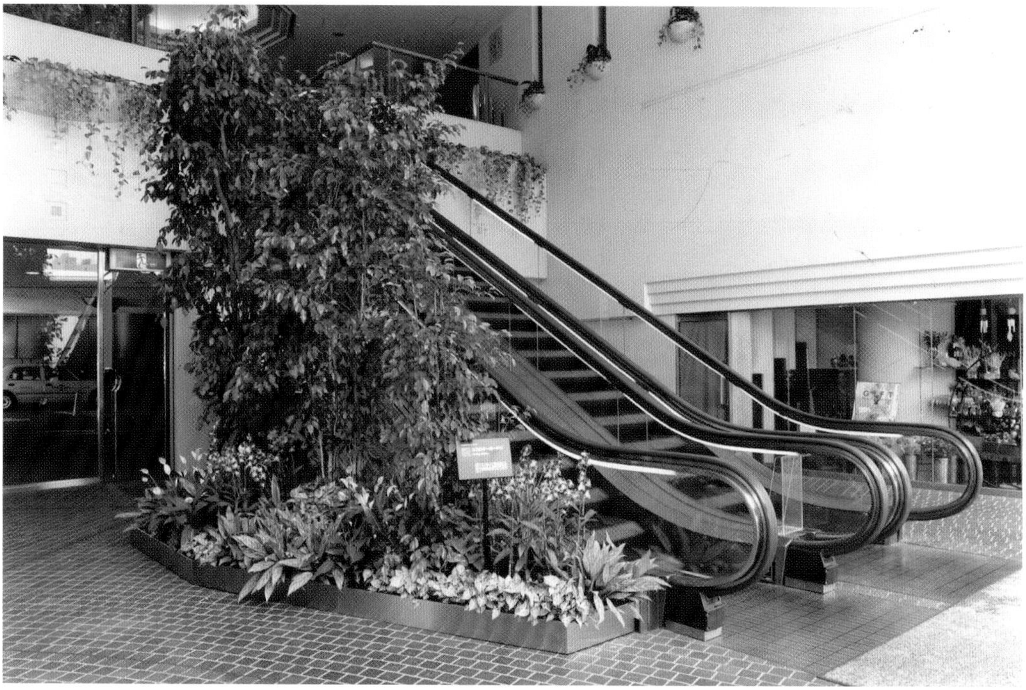

FIG. 3.5

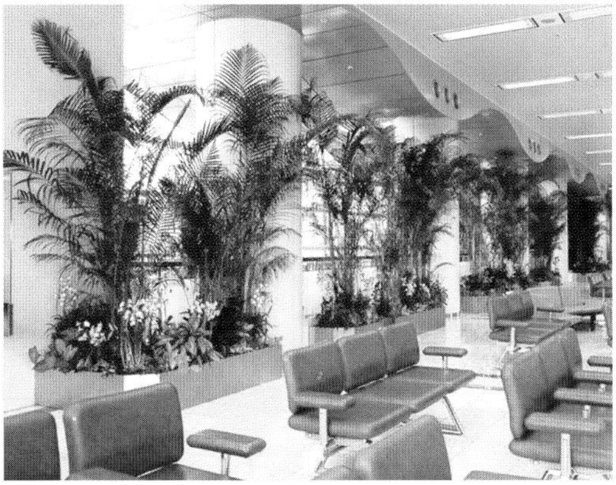

FIG. 3.6

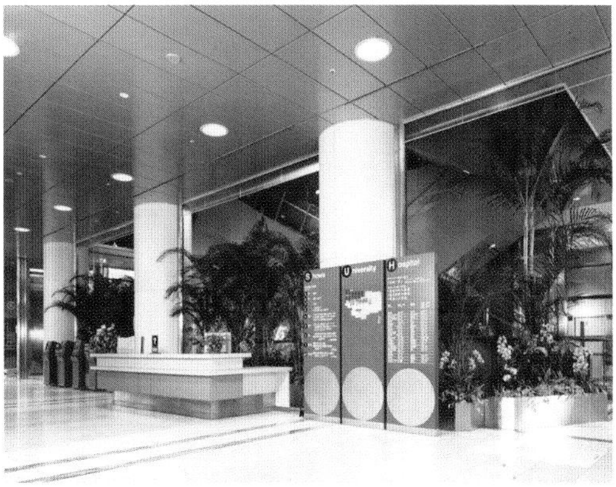

FIG. 3.7

regular guests although their cost is more expensive than rooms without a garden view (Fig. 3.9).

Embassy Suites Hotels have also found that large plant-filled atriums create a tranquil and relaxing atmosphere for their guests whether they are staying for business or pleasure. In fact, Embassy Suites requires that 50 per cent of each hotel atrium contain live plants and water elements, such as waterfalls and streams, and 20 per cent of the decorative railings overlooking the atrium must incorporate living plant life. Other hotels, such as Hyatt, also make use of lush garden settings to attract guests to their location.

The interior plant industry has seen an increased demand by the public for more plants indoors. There is now an entire profession, horticultural therapy, devoted to the healing power of plants. It recognizes the curative value of gardening and how it soothes the spirit, feeds the imagination and improves physical and mental well-being.

Humans depend upon the process of living plants for their existence on earth. Therefore, if we are to live predominantly inside energy-efficient buildings, we should bring plants, our life support system, inside with us. Unfortunately, the building industry has been slow to accept the role of plants in creating a healthy environment for people to live and work. This is primarily because architects and building engineers are not trained in the health benefits derived from being near plants. Their training generally centres on mechanical ventilation as a means of getting fresh air inside buildings. The overwhelming evidence demonstrating the health value of interior plants may eventually compel the building industry to consider designing plants into tightly sealed

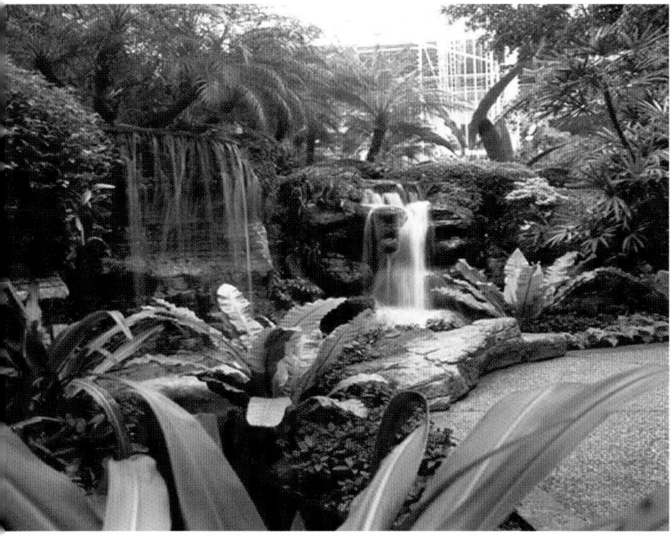

FIG. 3.8

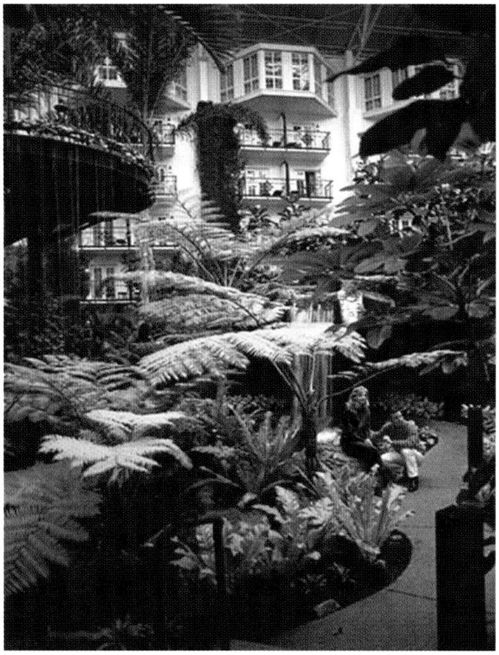

FIG. 3.9

buildings to act as the air-purifying lungs of the building.

Office Buildings

In today's corporate world, more emphasis has begun to be placed on creating a more pleasant and comfortable work environment. Environmentally conscious corporate designers and facility managers are finally making employee health and comfort a priority. The benefits that result include higher employee satisfaction, reduced absenteeism, higher employee retention rates and the ability to better recruit new employees (Figs. 3.10 and 3.11).

Interior plantings in main lobbies and atriums have been common for many years. Yet, in the workspaces and offices throughout the building little thought was given to enhancing the workspace with live plants. Many misinformed or unaware management teams often look first to trimming their 'plant budget' whenever operating budgets are tight. Yet, studies show that the positive effects plants have on employee perception, job satisfaction and morale far outweigh the cost. Outsourcing interior plantings to professional interior-scapers is a wise investment. These professionals have the expertise to design, install and maintain the company's plant investment. A Gallop poll's results state that two-thirds of the American workforce list gardening as their favourite hobby. Maybe this helps to explain the rise in employee morale when plants are present around them.

Relative Humidity and Human Comfort

Relative humidity is the amount of moisture present in the surrounding air and usually expressed as a percentage of the maximum amount the air has the capacity to hold. The generally accepted range for human comfort is between 30 and 60 per cent.

Relative humidity, as it relates to human health and well-being in the indoor environment, has only recently gained importance. Two factors are significant in raising awareness: 1) The fact that many in our modern society may spend as much as 90 per cent of their time indoors; and 2) As building envelopes are sealed more tightly for energy conservation, indoor air quality issues are of major concern.

The relative humidity of the air inside buildings, especially when heated during winter months, can be extremely low. Without supplemental moisture, the relative humidity decreases as air is heated. In hot humid climates, indoor air is cooled by mechanical air conditioning. During this process, condensation collects on the cooling coils. This collected water is then drained into the building's plumbing system rather than adding the moisture back to the conditioned air. As a result, even in hot summer months, a building's humidity level may be below the range of human comfort. Most buildings do not have systems in place that humidify the air within acceptable ranges. In those buildings that do humidify the air, many have experienced that humidifiers become contaminated with disease-causing micro-organisms.

In urban areas, it is estimated that more than 80 per cent of all diseases are produced by viruses and other micro-organisms

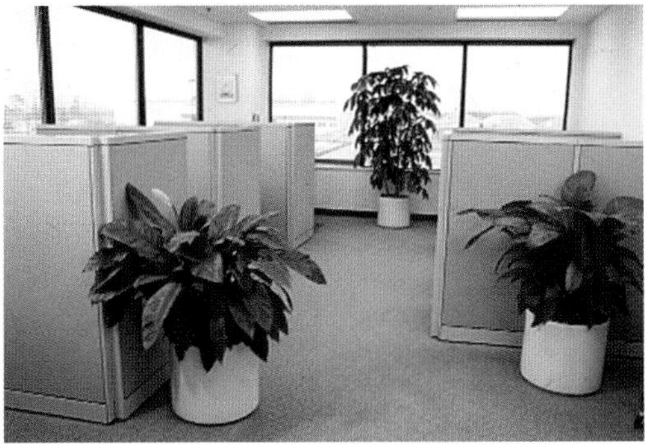

FIG. 3.10

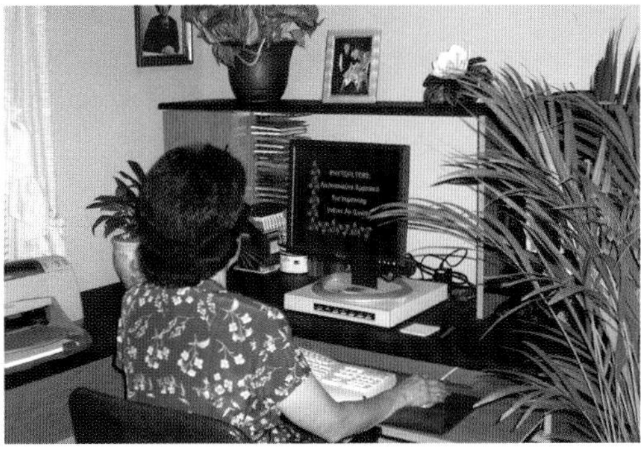

FIG. 3.11

entering the body through the respiratory system. Dry air not only dries the skin but also dries the mucus membrane lining which helps protect the respiratory system from harmful microbes and particulates. When the membranes become dry, viruses present in the ambient air can more easily enter the lungs. The lungs are a moist environment and harbour a perfect place for viruses to become activated, producing colds, influenza and other illnesses.

When relative humidity is too high, numerous problems can occur. Moisture may condensate on cold surfaces, including windows and exterior walls. These places become harbingers for many moulds and mildews. Allergic diseases like asthma and rhinitis can be triggered by either too high or too low relative humidity.

In general, studies show that relative humidity (rh) has the following effects:

- Bacteria increase at 30 per cent or less and 60 per cent or more rh.
- Viruses increase at 50 per cent or less and 70 per cent or more rh.
- Fungi increases at 60 per cent or more rh.
- Mites increase at 50 per cent or more rh.
- Respiratory infections increase at 50 per cent or less and unknown above 50 per cent rh.
- Asthma difficulties increase at either less than or higher than 50 per cent rh.
- Chemical interactions increase at 30 per cent or more rh.
- Ozone production increases at 75 per cent or less rh.

More recent studies have sought to determine the effect plants play on humidity in the indoor environment. Plants naturally reduce transpiration rates when the humidity is high and increase transpiration rates when the humidity is low. Plants do this in an effort to maintain humidity within their comfort zone. Luckily for us humans, interior plants thrive within the same relative humidity range (30 to 60 per cent) that is the most healthful for humans.

RELATIVE HUMIDITY LEVELS

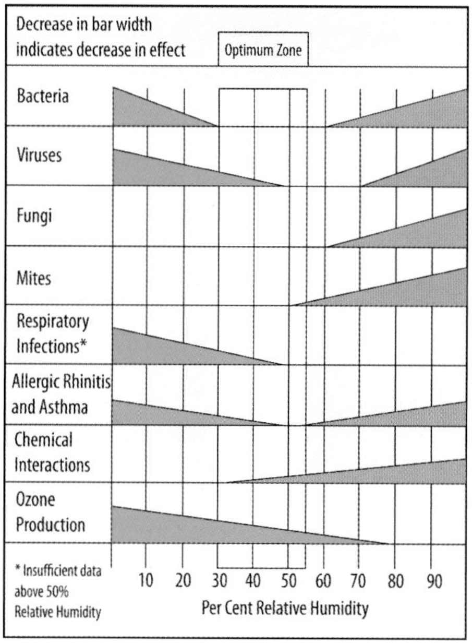

Source: ASHRAE Transactions, 1985, Vol. 91, Part I

A crossover study conducted by Dr Tové Fjeld in Norway sought to quantify the measurable effects of plants on office workers. The study was conducted in fifty-one offices. All participants worked in identical single offices. When plants were present, the office workers were exposed to thirteen commonly used interior foliage plants within the 10 sq m floor area. The table below shows some of the data the study produced.

HEALTH IMPROVEMENTS AFTER THE INTRODUCTION OF INTERIOR PLANTS

Symptom	Health Improvement %
Fatigue	32% less
Headache	45% less
Sore/dry throats	22% less
Coughs	38% less
Dry facial skin	11% less

The results indicated an overall average of 23 per cent lower incidence of twelve common symptoms when plants were present. Nearly identical results were verified by Dr Fjeld when measuring the effects of indoor plants together with full-spectrum fluorescent lighting on health and discomfort symptoms among personnel working in a hospital radiology department. Workers who spent most of their day in the room showed a 34 per cent decrease in complaints, while workers spending less than 40 per cent of their day in the room had only a 17 per cent decrease in complaints.

Dr Virginia Lohr, a Washington State University professor, conducted a four-month study (between December and March) to determine interior plants' influence on relative humidity both in the presence and absence of plants in a single office space within a building having a HVAC system. The study showed that in the presence of plants, relative humidity increased and stabilized within the human comfort range. Without plants, the humidity level dipped slightly below the recommended range.

Negative Air Ions

Negative ions are charged airborne particles that are formed when enough energy acts on a molecule, such as water, to eject an electron. The displaced electron attaches itself to a nearby molecule that becomes a negative ion.

In nature, negative ions are formed in a variety of ways: UV light, airflow friction, lightning, falling water and by plants. Plant leaves produce negative ions as they emit water vapour. Plants that have the highest transpiration rates can be expected to produce the most number of negative ions. Waterfalls and tropical forests create large numbers of negative ions.

The ability of plants to produce negative ions is a phenomenon that has been accepted by most for decades. The air we breathe contains both positive and negative ions. Studies have demonstrated that the ratio of positively to negatively charged molecules can have marked biological effects on plants and animals. Ion balance that favours positively charged ions may play a significant role in a wide range of human ailments, including respiratory infections in office workers and the malaise caused by weather conditions. Further, artificially generated air ions may prove valuable as a therapeutic modality in the treatment of certain diseases. The question remains whether artificially produced negative ions have the same psychological effects on people as naturally occurring ions.

Physicians and environmental scientists have long suspected that the detrimental effects of 'stagnant air' in crowded rooms were due to ion depletion. In 1939, Japanese scientists, S. Kimura, M. Ashiba and L. Matushima showed that if temperature, humidity and carbon dioxide levels were all kept within a comfort range, but the ion level was reduced, individuals suffered discomfort and depression. These symptoms were promptly relieved when normal ion densities were restored by the use of ion generators. It is now possible to make available highly beneficial ion-rich microenvironments that go hand in hand with efforts to reduce the air pollutants responsible for diminishing the amount of negative ions in the indoor environment. Toshiba Home Technology Corporation sells fans and dehumidifiers with negative ion features. Refrigerators, air conditioners and other products are also marketed in Japan that release negative ions into the indoor environments.

Studies by the US Department of Agriculture (USDA) have demonstrated the bactericidal effects of negative ions on airborne and surface bacterial contamination. An aerosol containing the bacterium *Salmonella enteritidis* was pumped into a sealed plastic chamber containing plates of bacterial growth agar attached to the walls, and the top and bottom of the chamber. The chamber was exposed to the aerosol for three hours with and without exposure to high levels of negative ions. An average greater than 10,000 cfu/plate was observed on plates exposed to the aerosol without high levels of negative ions (a control) and compared with an average of less than 53 cfu/plate exposed to high levels of negative ions.

Another small chamber study was conducted to determine the effect of negative ions on a bacterial culture mix collected from a poultry processing facility. The mixed bacterial population was grown on stainless steel coupons of 0.4 x 1.57 inches (1 x 4 cm) and attached to the base of the test chamber. Negative ions effectively decreased the survival level of bacteria on stainless steel with a reduction of 99.8 per cent. These results indicate that high levels of negative air ions can significantly reduce the level of bacteria both in the air and on surfaces.

Interior landscape companies such as Takenaka Garden Afforestation, Inc. advocate the use of ecology gardens for improving the quality of air in modern buildings. Many studies have shown that interior plants can remove VOCs that accumulate in tightly sealed buildings and reduce the numbers of moulds and other microbes in the air surrounding plant leaves. Although the mechanism used by plants to reduce airborne microbes is not known, it is believed that negative ions play a major role in this process.

Recent studies by Dr Tomoo Ryushi, Department of Human Physiology, Tokyo Metropolitan University and Takenaka Garden Afforestation, Inc., demonstrated that the density of negative air ions in a room free of plants was as low as 9 to 12 cubic inches (150 to 200/ cubic cm), but when areca palms and peace lily were added to the room negative ions increased to a level of 60 cubic inches (1,000/ cubic cm) within twenty-four hours. UV light is also used in conjunction with living plants to increase the air purifying properties of planter systems.

SUMMARY

Science has now offered definitive proof to bolster what we have always known instinctively – that humans benefit from a close association with nature. Today's trend toward a more holistic approach to the spaces where we reside and work is beneficial to our health and well-being.

We can rest assured that placing interior plants within built spaces helps to soothe and calm our senses, purify and refresh the air we breathe and add beneficial moisture and negative ions to our environment. In general, if plants are healthy and thriving indoors, then we might safely assume that the space is a healthy environment for us as well.

We are naturally attracted to plantings of lush, living greenery, whether indoors or in green spaces within congested cities of concrete and steel. We enjoy the calm, tranquil setting and benefit physically, mentally and spiritually from the respite of our otherwise harried, busy lives. The availability of lush greenery, flowering plants and even trees meets an essential human need. In our modern society where time is spent predominantly indoors, we must surround ourselves with living plants for their health-giving benefits.

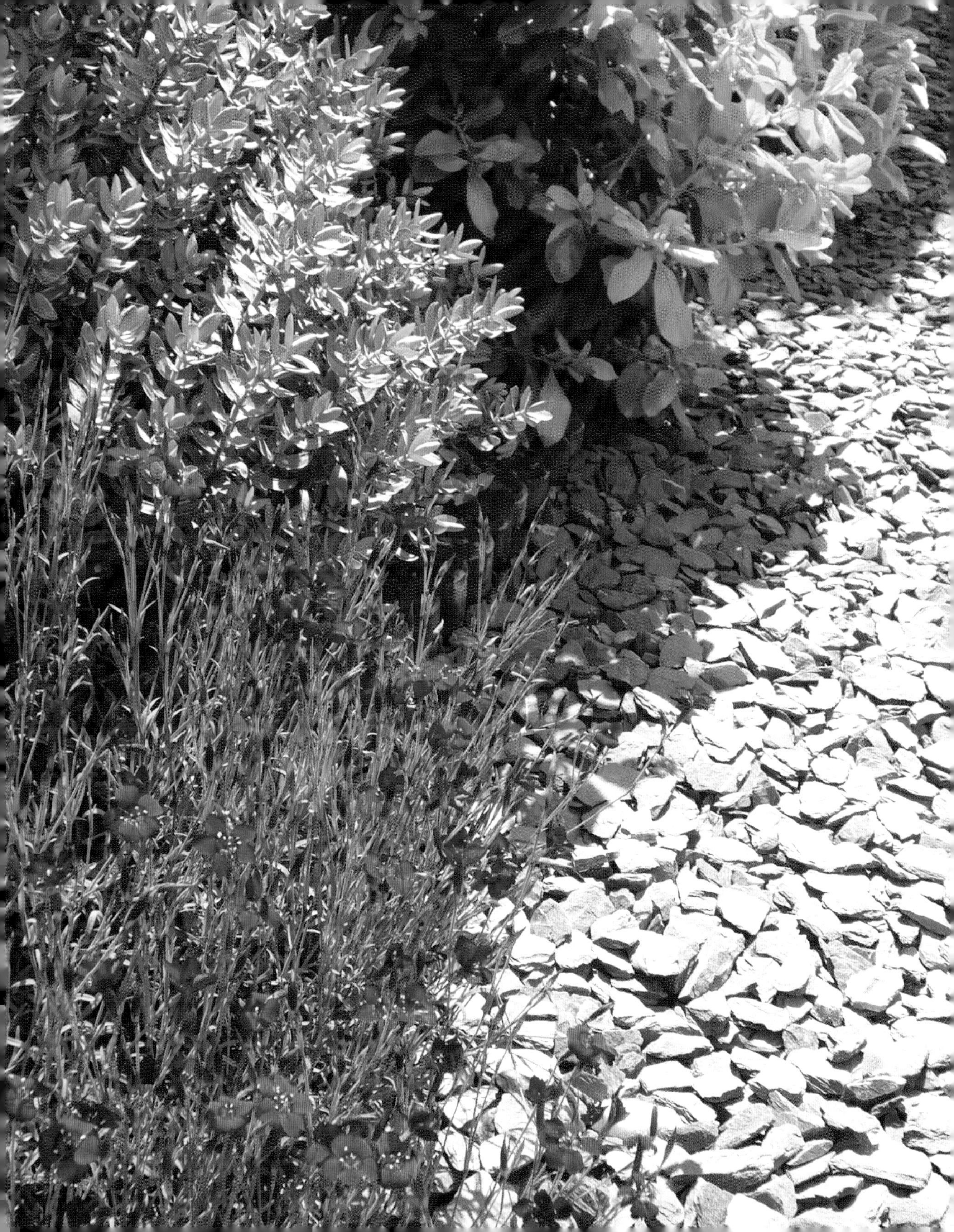

Gardening

Gardens are as old as civilization itself. The word garden is derived from the Anglo Saxon word *gyrdon*, meaning to *enclose*. Horticulture is a branch of agriculture relating to garden crops, primarily fruits, vegetables or ornamental plants. The word derives its name from the Latin *hortus*, meaning 'garden' and *colere*, meaning 'to cultivate'. Horticulture usually refers to intensive commercial production of garden crops. Gardening, on the other hand, generally refers to the laying out and care of a parcel of land that is used at least in part for the cultivation of plants such as herbs, fruits, vegetables or flowers. The garden began as an enclosure for vegetables or fruit trees and was usually situated near the house. It was enclosed with a hedge, fence or wall to keep out animals or thieves. Gardens range in size from a small container-grown garden on a private balcony or patio to large public gardens. In its art form, gardening focuses on the arrangement of plants that is both aesthetically pleasing to the human eye and is in harmony with its surroundings. On a scientific plane, gardening is concerned with the principles and techniques of plant cultivation.

There are many varieties of garden styles that are dictated by their layout, location and plant species. Design and colour are two important elements of a beautiful and functional garden. The microclimate within a given space often dictates the garden style and functional layout. Yet, a private garden is limited only by the imagination of its owner within the limits of climate, materials and resources.

Garden types usually fall within the following categories: 1) flower gardens, 2) woodland gardens, 3) rock gardens, 4) water gardens, 5) herb and vegetable gardens, and 6) speciality gardens, such as roof gardens or scented gardens. On a large scale, a garden might encompass several or all of the various garden types.

The most obvious benefits of gardening are the production of fresh fruits and vegetables or the sheer pleasure of viewing beautiful flowering and foliage plants and the wildlife gardens attract, such as birds and butterflies. It is not difficult to see that gardening is also a healthy pastime. The obvious benefit to one's personal health is the physical activity gardening entails. Most people who live in a modern, urban environment have little opportunity to be outdoors. Just getting outside to enjoy activities such as gardening relieves stress from our frenzied lives. Cultivating soil and connecting with nature can also lower blood pressure, cut cholesterol, build muscles and fight depression.

Gardening has become the number one leisure activity in the United States and Canada, even surpassing sports. A closer observation reveals other less obvious benefits that have made this activity so popular. Gardening provides a venue for creativity and can be mentally stimulating. A garden setting may also offer a quiet location for self-reflection and meditation or a peaceful atmosphere for activities such as Tai Chi or yoga. These are traditional forms of Chinese and Indian mind/body exercises and meditation techniques that use slow sets of body movements and controlled breathing. They are done to improve balance, flexibility, muscle strength and overall health. However, simply relaxing and enjoying nature's wonders in a peaceful garden setting can contribute to better health in general.

A basic understanding of botany can be attained by simply learning more about the plants that you grow whether they are flowers, foliage, fruits or vegetables. Sharing your gardening interests and ideas with other enthusiasts affords the opportunity to cultivate new friendships.

In an urban environment, gardens and landscaping contribute significantly to the improvement of air quality, the lowering of temperatures during summer months, and the interaction of city-dwellers with nature. Simply relaxing and enjoying nature's wonders in a peaceful garden setting can contribute to better health. Studies have shown that women of age fifty and older who gardened at least once a week had higher bone density than those who jogged, walked, swam or did aerobics. Gardening can also produce an increase in endorphins similar to those experienced when jogging and cycling. No matter how simple the garden, even if it is only a couple of container-grown plants, it can still provide one with a wealth of enjoyment and pleasure.

Western Gardens

When one considers historic Western gardens, one immediately thinks of Great Britain. Oxford University's Botanic Garden is the oldest, founded in 1621. This botanic garden probably contains more biological diversity than any other two-hectare plot on earth. Originally, the garden was divided into four parts to receive plant specimens brought back by explorers to the four continents – Europe, Asia, Africa and America. It was set up by Henry Danvers, Earl of Danby, for the advancement of medicine and the promotion of learning. Today, the garden seeks to remind its visitors that our food and drink, many of our medicines and much of our clothing and building materials come from plants. In fact, our very existence is reliant upon plants to provide us with the air we breathe.

The Chelsea Physic Garden in Chelsea, England, was founded in 1673 by the Worshipful Company of Apothecaries and is England's second oldest botanic garden. Its purpose was to promote the study of botany for medicinal purposes, known at that time as 'physic' or healing arts and to train apprentices in identifying plants. The historic gardens of England still retain their importance.

The Bonn University Botanic Garden, one of the oldest and most traditional gardens north of the Alps, goes back more than 400 years. The existence of a castle and a simple garden is first recorded in a drawing dated 1578. The total area of the garden is 14.82 acres (6 hectares) of which greenhouses occupy 0.62 acres (0.25 hectares). The

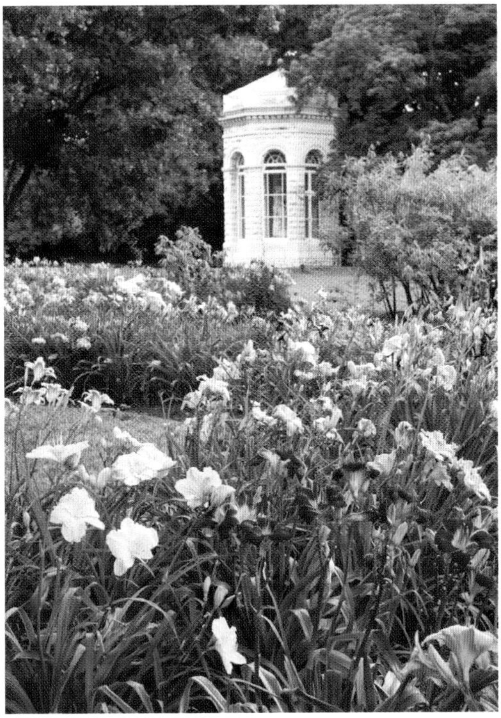

FIG. 4.1

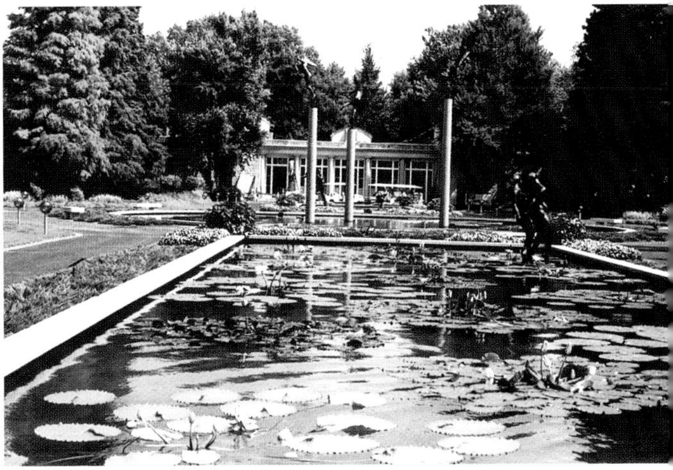

FIG. 4.2

botanical garden is one of the university's scientific institutions. In addition, the garden is open to school classes and individual students, young and old. The garden is also a place to relax in a busy centre of Bonn, Germany. These are only a few examples of the oldest of numerous botanical gardens located throughout Europe.

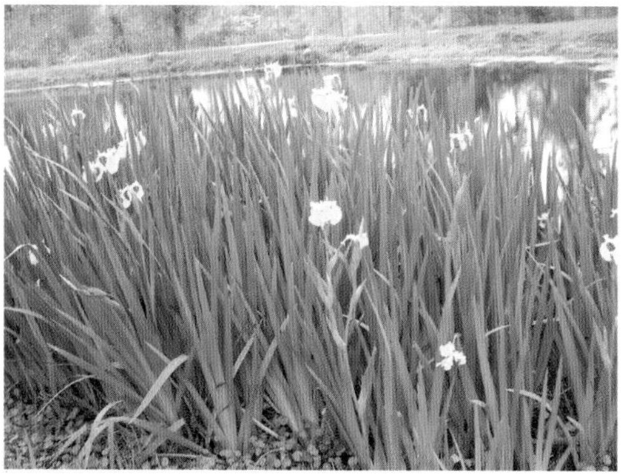

Fig. 4.3

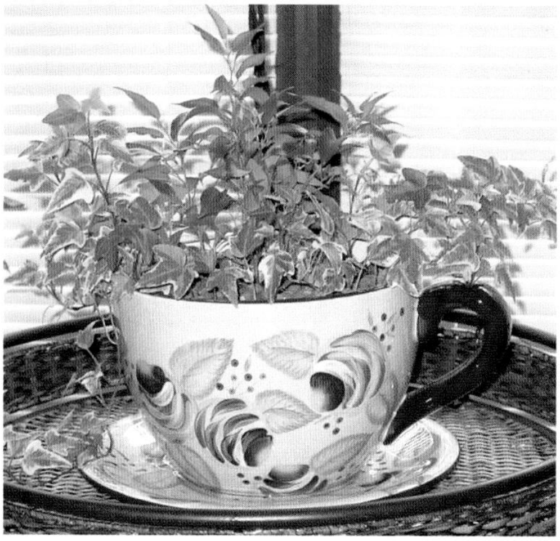

FIG. 4.4

The Missouri Botanical Gardens located in St Louis, Missouri, is one of America's oldest botanical gardens (Figs. 4.1, 4.2 and 4.6). Another of America's botanical gardens that can trace its beginnings to 1816 is the United States Botanical Gardens located in Washington, DC. Botanical gardens, public gardens, arboretums and national and state parks are very popular in America and are located throughout the States. These areas provide a tremendous diversity of plant and animal life and are available for all to enjoy.

However, not all gardens have formal designs. The varying shapes, sizes and forms of gardens are as diverse as their caretakers.

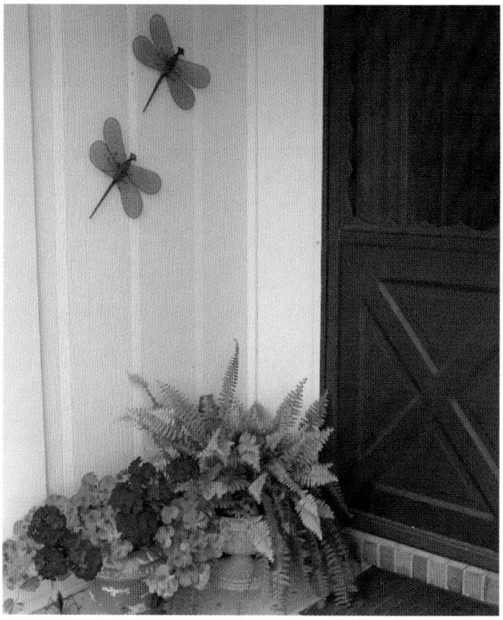

FIG. 4.5

Almost everyone grows some kind of plants, whether it is a small pot of herbs on a windowsill, a large welcoming planter at the front entrance or extensive landscaping around the perimeter of one's home. We are all gardeners of some kind. Even those dwelling deep within concrete jungles can enjoy public green spaces, parks or interior plantings in public buildings. The boundaries of one's garden are limited only by the imagination.

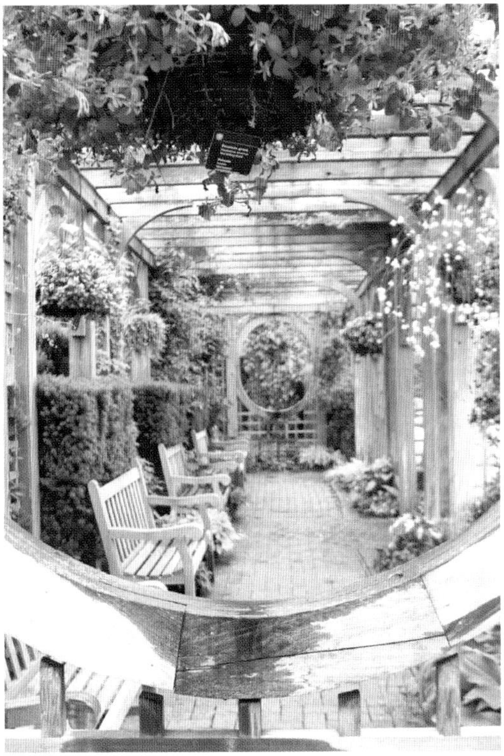

FIG. 4.6

Japanese Gardens

Japanese gardens have developed over many centuries. They represent a different approach to nature than Western gardens. However, all gardens are shaped by religious and philosophical beliefs. Western gardens are predominantly influenced by Christianity, while Japanese gardens are rooted in Shintoism, Hinduism, Taoism and Buddhism. Japanese gardens are designed to restore inner calm and peace of mind. Nature, plants and gardens are very important to Japanese culture and reflect the beliefs of both Shintoism and Buddhism.

The fundamentals of Japanese garden design stem from four principles that are connected to Shintoism. The garden must: 1) create a likeness to the natural world; 2) follow the natural contour of the land; 3) be asymmetrical or off-balanced and irregular; and 4) try to capture the spirit or feeling of the location.

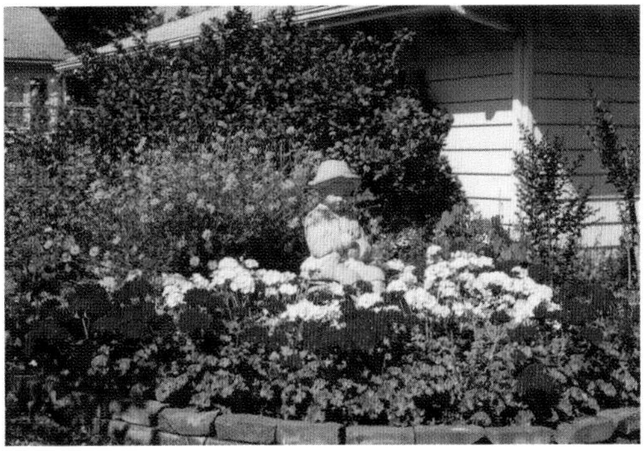

FIG. 4.7

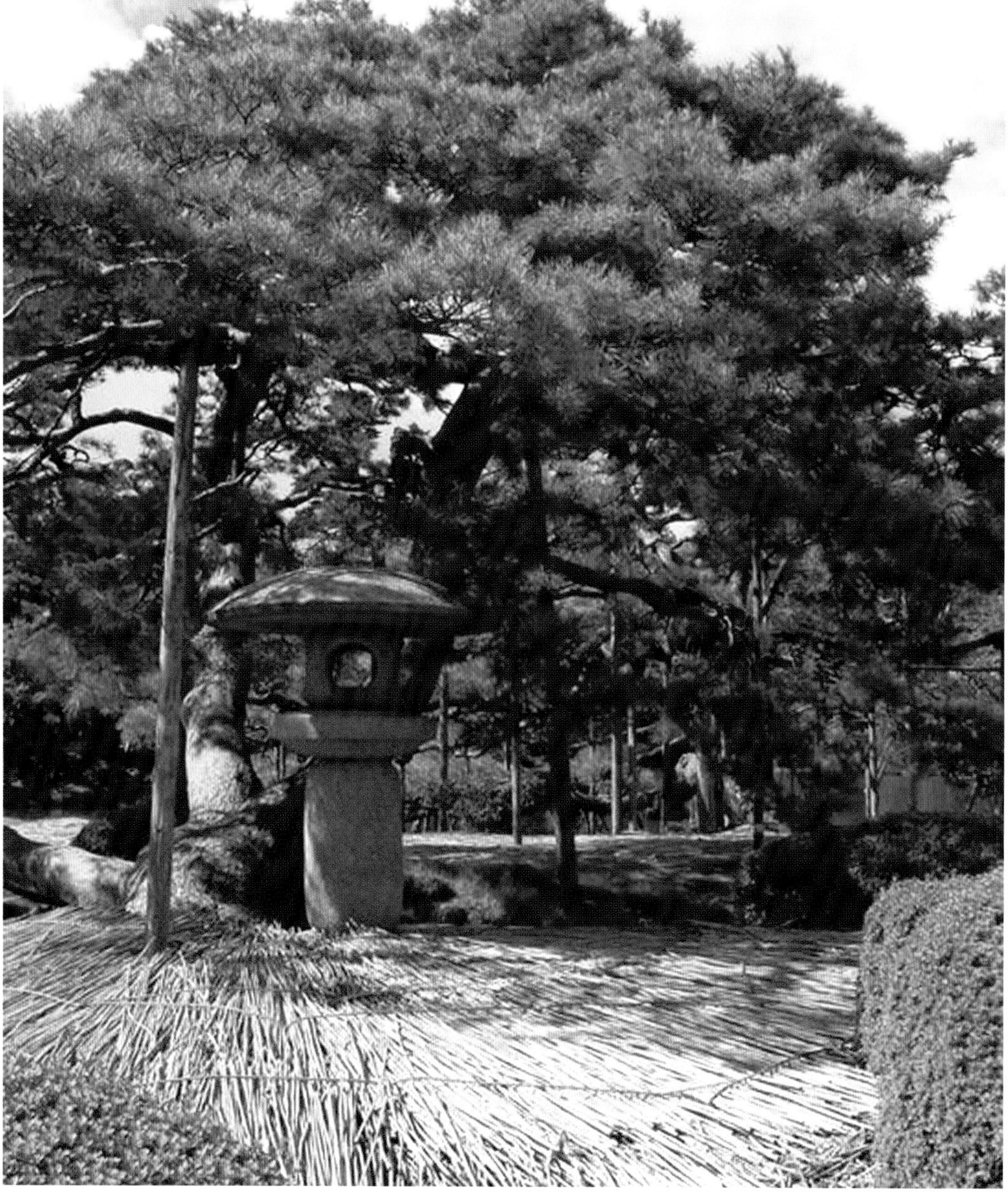

FIG. 4.8

The aim of a Japanese garden is to seek harmony with nature, thereby showing strong appreciation for natural elements such as water, trees and rocks. Trees and stones are grouped in odd numbers. This design element is rooted in the religious belief that evil spirits walk in straight lines. Thus, evil spirits can be warded off by the creation of winding, twisted paths.

In the Japanese garden there are no showy beds of colourful flowers that are typical of a Western garden. Blooming plants lack the permanence that water, trees, shrubs and stones have. Aged trees, often with a small sign depicting their age, are common elements in Japanese gardens (Fig. 4.8). Placement of plants is extremely important to the point of even determining how the plant's reflection will appear in a nearby water element. Water is a vital element in the garden. In fact, the Japanese word for gardener means 'He who makes

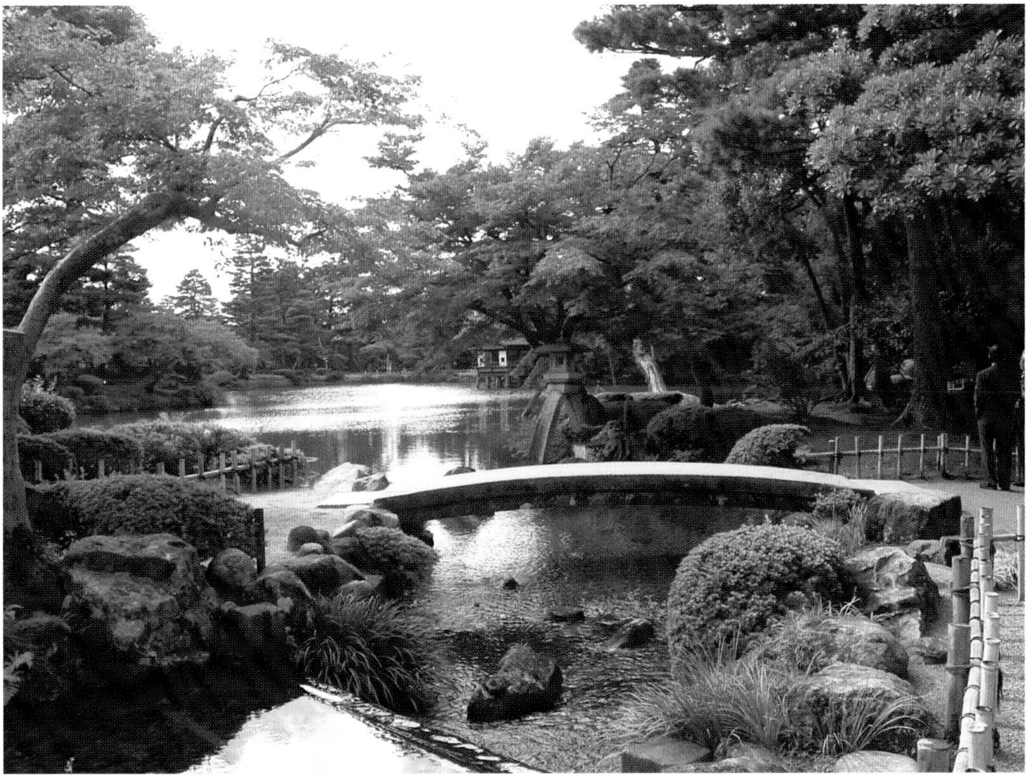

FIG. 4.9

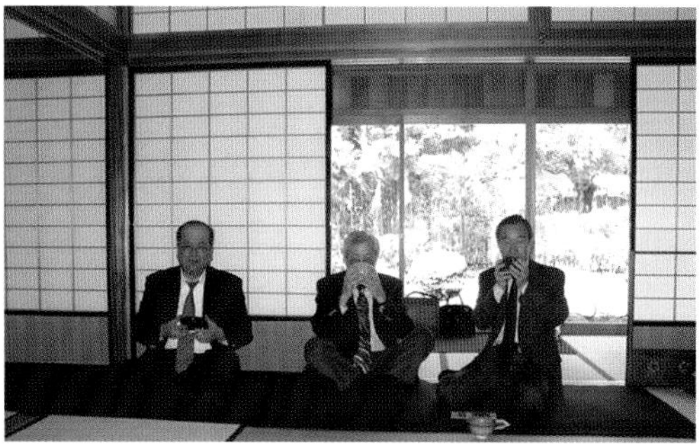

FIG. 4.10

the bed of streams'. Other important elements are stone, gravel and bamboo. The typical Japanese garden has some type of element that demarcates it from the surrounding land, whether it is through fencing or stones or trees to create a border.

Japanese garden design ensures that every detail is chosen for a reason. One must study the design carefully to fully comprehend the role of garden elements: rocks represent mountains; lanterns represent temples; bushes become trees; and ponds represent lakes, seas and oceans.

Zen rock gardens are also popular 'dry gardens'. They consist of sand, rock and stone and provide a place for quiet reflection and contemplation. These gardens were originally developed in the fifteenth century by Buddhist monks. Sand represented the ocean and stones represented gods, mountains and animals. The sand was carefully raked to represent waves upon the ocean. Zen rock gardens are popular today in many societies.

Kairakuen in Ibaraki Prefecture, Kenrokuen in Ishikawa Prefecture and Kourakuen in Okayama Prefecture are generally recognized as Japan's three most beautiful landscape gardens. These gardens make use of broad expanses. Located in crowded cities, all three are popular public parks as well. The Kenrokuen Garden (Fig. 4.9) was once an expansive outer garden of Kanazawa Castle, a private garden of the ruling Maeda family, and constructed over a period of nearly two centuries. It did not become a public garden until 1871. Kenrokuen Garden makes use of ponds, streams, waterfalls, bridges, teahouses, trees, stones and flowers. Water for the water elements in the park continues to flow from a river through a water system built in 1632.

Many Japanese gardens contain teahouses where visitors can partake in the traditional tea ceremony (Fig. 4.10). The teahouse is simple, austere and based upon a traditional farmhouse. There is typically an inner garden that is a private garden and is to be viewed only from the teahouse. This inner garden is a place for quiet reflection and peaceful solitude.

Roof Gardens

Green roofs, as one might expect, are plantings that are placed on the roof of a building. Green roofs have been in existence since ancient times. In fact, the Hanging Gardens of Babylon, one of the Seven Wonders of the Ancient World, did not actually 'hang' but were really roof gardens laid out in a series of raised terraces. These lush gardens were thought to have been built by King Nebuchadnezzar II about 600 BC and were located in what is now Babil province near Baghdad in Iraq.

Sod roofs were developed in Norway but used extensively by Scandinavians during ancient times. It is a type of roof covered with sod (a section of grass-covered top soil held together by matted roots) on top of several layers of birch bark on gently sloping roof boards. This thick roof was developed primarily as an affordable means of thermally insulating buildings. Birch is common in Northern Europe and is strong, water-resistant and soil-resistant. Sod roofs are still used as protection against extremely cold winters in Scandinavian countries, especially in Norway.

Over a century ago, Germany built green roofs primarily for fire protection. Early twentieth century architects like Le Corbusier and Frank Lloyd Wright envisioned 'gardens in the sky' in their urban plans. The development of contemporary green roof technology originated in Germany more than thirty years ago. Today, green roofs are employed by those seeking to be more environmentally responsible, especially in congested urban areas.

Germany has emerged as the world's leader in green roof design and installation. Industry estimates are that 10 per cent of all German roofs are greened. There are many cities in Europe that require or provide incentives for green roof regulations. The city of Stuttgart, Germany, now mandates a green roof for any new flat-roofed industrial building. However, in Asia, Japan is leading the way. In fact, Tokyo has been the first city to institute regulations requiring that 20 per cent of all new construction include green roofs.

Roof gardens offer many ecological benefits. They can help to offset the 'urban heat island effect'. According to Green Roofs for Healthy Cities, this is the difference in temperature between a city and the surrounding countryside. Urban areas contain up to 90 per cent hard surfaces such as rooftops and pavements. Hard and reflective surfaces absorb solar radiation and re-radiate it as heat. Plants, through the process of evapotranspiration, are able to cool the ambient temperature. During this process, plants use heat energy from their surroundings when evaporating water. On an annual basis, 10.76 sq ft (1 sq m) of foliage can evaporate up to 185 gallons (700 litres) of water.

Storm water runoff from hard surfaces flows through city drainage systems into

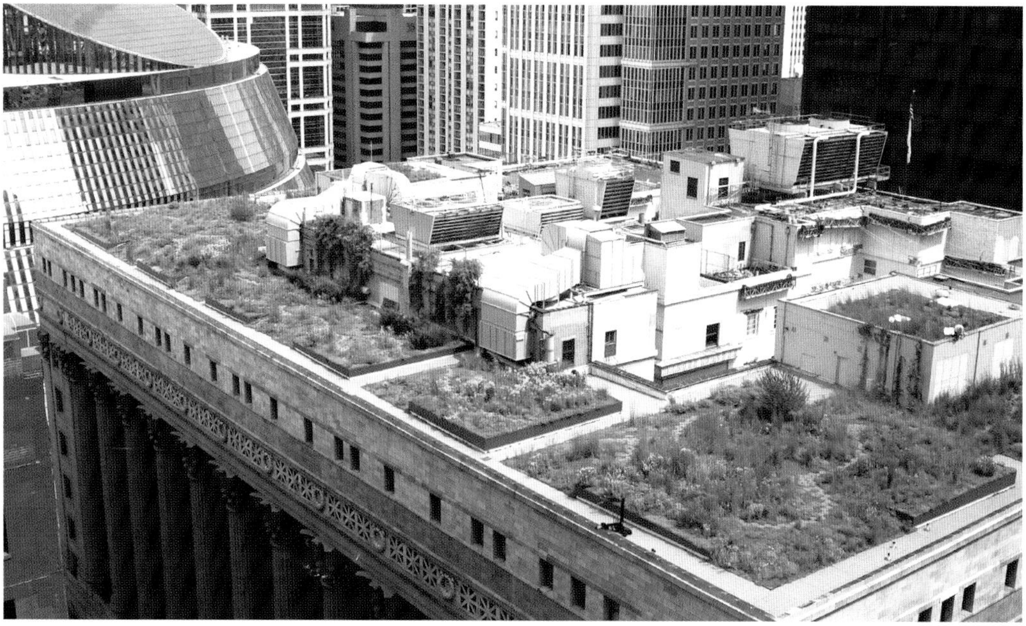

FIG. 4.11

receiving waters and is a major source of water pollution. Green roofs offer a method of reducing or delaying the volume of water and relieve the pressure on an overburdened drainage system, especially following a rainstorm. Plants and their planting media absorb rainwater, filter impurities and slowly release it into the drainage system. Depending upon the thickness of the vegetation, runoff can be reduced by as much as 50 per cent.

As plants transpire, they release moisture into the air helping to cool and humidify the microclimate of the roof. Plants and their growth media also aid by absorbing sound and providing thermal insulation. Landscaped roofs create natural habitats that attract more wildlife, such as birds and butterflies, to the urban area.

There are some drawbacks to green roofs, however. Foremost is safety. Engineers must insure that roofs are structurally sound and can bear the added weight of a roof garden. With increased use of lightweight plant growth media, most modern roofs can support the added 10 to 15 pounds (4.55 to 6.82 kg) wet weight per square foot. Maintenance is also a consideration and must be addressed for the roof garden to function properly. In the US, there are no strict guidelines for green roofs. A

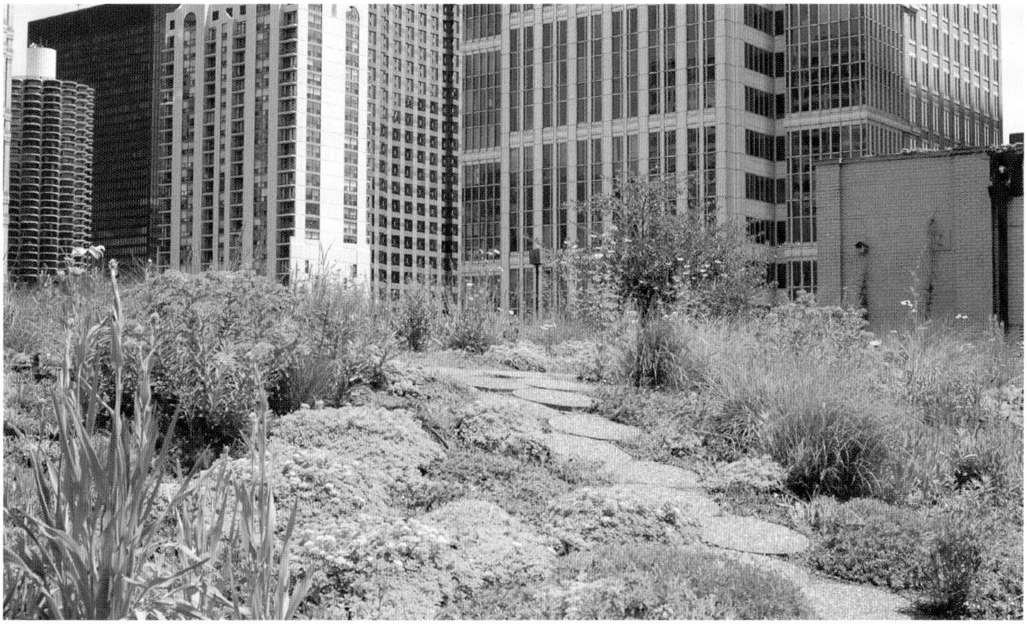

FIG. 4.12

standardizing of the technology must be implemented before rapid growth can be expected.

Although green roof technology has been slow to develop in the US, there are some significant projects throughout the country. Five roof gardens were installed atop the seventh floor of New York City's Rockefeller Center between 1933 and 1936. These gardens were built for their aesthetic value, especially for tenants having a view from nearby high-rise buildings. These gardens continue to enhance the view today.

The famous Kaiser Center roof garden located in Oakland, California, was inspired by the Rockefeller Center roof gardens. Edgar Kaiser, son of the empire's founder, had worked in offices in New York City that looked out over the Rockefeller Center roof gardens, the first major roof garden in the US. This inspired him to build one of the largest roof gardens in the world in 1960. The Kaiser roof garden was designed by landscape architect, Theodore Osmundson. It encompasses 2.96 acres (1.2 hectares) of green space across the connected roofs of three buildings, a block from Oakland's Lake Merritt.

Chicago is a leading proponent of roof garden technology. The Chicago City Hall maintains a roof garden atop its eleven-storey office building (Figs. 4.11 and 4.12). Constructed in 2000, the garden initially began as a demonstration project. As a part of the City's Urban Heat Island Initiative, the project sought to determine the benefits of roof gardens, in particular, their effect on temperature and air quality within their microclimate. The garden consists of 20,000 plants of more than 150 species, including shrubs, vines and trees. Most plants are prairie plants, such as sedum, and Mediterranean plants that are drought tolerant and can withstand wind. The garden attracts crickets, butterflies, birds and even has beehives to house an active bee colony.

According to Chief Environmental Officer Sadhu Johnston, Chicago Department of Environment, a roof garden provides four main benefits: 1) beauty, 2) storm water retention, 3) urban heat island effect, and 4) a longer lasting roof. Leading by example, the city has a vibrant programme to encourage the expansion of roof garden technology, especially within its downtown area.

In June 2002, Toyota established Sichuan Toyota Nitan Development Co. Ltd., in Chengdu, Sichuan Province, China. The company specializes in mining, processing and export of the Yuexi peat which has excellent water and nutrient retention properties. Toyota has determined that this peat is ideal for use in roof gardening projects in Japan. In December 2001, Toyota had established Toyota Roof Garden Corporation in Japan for the purpose of promoting Yuexi peat use in the roof garden business.

While roof gardens are attractive and ecologically beneficial, they offer many other beneficial functions as well. A roof garden can extend the life of roofs, cut air conditioning and heating costs for buildings by providing insulation against winter cold and summer heat. It is estimated that green roofs can last up to twice as long as conventional roofs. A study by Environment Canada found that a typical one-storey building with a grass roof and 3.9 inches (10 cm) of growing medium would result in a 25 per cent reduction in summer cooling needs.

Roof gardens can take on many forms ranging from modular planters to a continuous layer of growth media and vegetation over the entire roof area. Most roof gardens that allow visitors utilize modular designs with walking paths and park benches. The number and species of plants that roof gardens can accommodate are, however, limited by climate, structural design and maintenance budgets. The planting media usually consists of lightweight expanded clay or shale pebbles, also commonly used in hydroponic growth systems (see Fig. 4.13).

As the production of green roofs and roof garden components increases, the cost for

PRINCIPAL GREEN ROOF TECHNOLOGY COMPONENTS

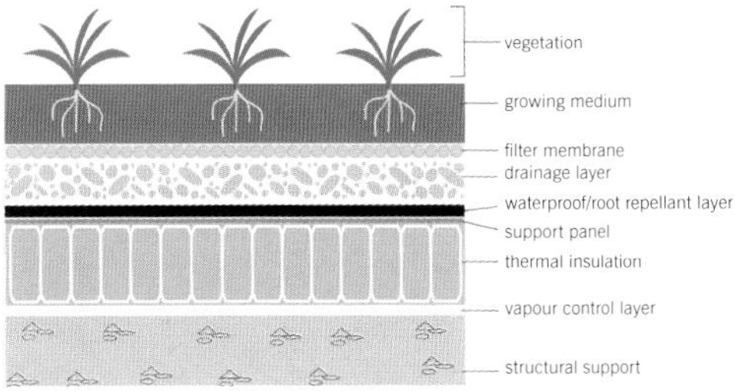

Source: National Research Council, Institute for Research in Construction

FIG. 4.13

these systems should decrease, making them affordable to more clients. As this eco-technology grows in popularity, it is inevitable that some designs will utilize roof gardens to develop a complete ecosystem for the building whereby plants can utilize human waste as a fertilizer, while purifying the wastewater. As the wastewater is purified, it can then be used to water other landscaping within the building perimeter, thus completing the recycling process. From almost any point of view, roof gardens are environmentally and economically viable options to bring an oasis of nature into urban areas.

Vegetable Gardening and Commercial Crop Production

Gardening is almost as old as humankind itself. From earliest recorded history there is evidence of efforts to cultivate plants for human sustenance. In earlier times, the successful yield of one's cultivation efforts often determined one's survival. At the very least, successfully harvesting produce meant the difference between feast and famine. In the twenty-first century, these pressures only hold true for those living in the poorest of countries. In most modern countries, fresh food is reliably available and affordable in nearby markets. Therefore, the need for each household to at least partially produce its own food is not significant.

People living in rural America grew most of their own food up until the late 1940s, using animal waste as fertilizer. By the early 1950s, large farm operations and food processors began to flood the market with inexpensive, processed foods. It quickly became more expensive to grow food in a backyard garden or on a family farm than to buy it at the supermarket. The convenience that supermarkets afforded a busy lifestyle resulted in a rapid shift from fresh homegrown vegetables to highly processed canned goods. Unfortunately, food prices are increasing throughout the world. Many factors affect food prices, including weather conditions, from floods to droughts; rising fuel and shipping costs; continued population growth; and the conversion of food crops to biofuels.

Water is essential for life and food production. However, it is not evenly distributed over the earth. Northern India averages more than 400 inches (10 m) per year while the northern region of Chile may not receive rain for several years. In large developed countries, such as the US, one region might experience drought conditions while another area is experiencing floods. Just such a scenario occurred in 2008. The world's population continues its steady rise with population estimates being as high as 8 billion by 2025. Humans are placing more and more stress on the limited supply of fresh water and affordable food.

Added to this burden is the increased production of biofuels from crops. The crops required for biofuels have a high content of sugar or starch, like sugarcane or corn. The US accounts for about 40 per cent of the world's total corn production and more than half of all corn exports. Greater demand for corn has yielded higher returns for farmers. So, farmers are planting more acres with corn and fewer acres with other staple crops, like wheat and rice. The surge in ethanol production too has led to higher prices for both processed and staple grains around the world. Those most impacted by higher food prices are residents of impoverished nations.

Shipping and fuel costs continue to rise as well. It is not uncommon for food to be grown in Western and Midwest states and shipped to the East Coast of the US. Of course, these costs are passed along to consumers. These factors have led to consumers considering the option of purchasing locally grown crops. Many are beginning to rethink how and where food is produced. With today's worldwide financial crisis, food shortages are a high possibility. Changing weather patterns are also causing crop failures in many countries. As a result, scientists are beginning to look at the feasibility of growing food crops in environmentally controlled facilities.

Some have proposed rooftop green houses atop supermarkets where fresh produce can be harvested and brought immediately into the supermarkets. This kind of produce would be fresher, more nutritious and cheaper. Food crops that have a faster rate of growth than indoor foliage plants produce more oxygen and remove more carbon dioxide. Therefore, the marriage of local food production and indoor air purification may prove to be an ideal combination. Space research has shown, through the development of 'closed ecological life-support systems' for future long-term space habitation, that this concept has great potential.

Universities and other scientists are exploring ways to produce food in urban settings. Environmental scientist, Dickson Despommier of Columbia University has proposed vertical farming within skyscrapers. His idea for a thirty-storey building could potentially provide 50,000 people with fruits, vegetables and chickens. Through the use of soil-free hydroponic farming, the conversion of sewage into electricity, climate-controlled environmental conditions and the elimination of high shipping costs could possibly yield more economical food production. Such concepts are only ideas as of yet. However, investors in Abu Dhabi and South Korea are considering their viability for new planned 'eco-cities'. While these concepts may or may not prove economically feasible, it is obvious that we will need new methods of producing food if the supply is to remain abundant and affordable.

Garden clubs in America focus their efforts almost exclusively on ornamental plants grown for their aesthetic value, not for food. Today, it is not food shortage that is detrimental to the health of people in highly developed countries, but the overabundance of highly processed foods laden with salt, sugar, synthetic chemicals and pesticides. The US currently ranks among the highest in the world in obesity and degenerative diseases, both of which have a direct correlation to diet and lifestyle. Thankfully, because of public awareness of the dangers to human health associated with synthetic chemicals in fertilizers and pesticides, a growing number of people around the world are beginning to return to the more natural approach of organic farming.

According to the US Department of Agriculture (USDA), certified organic agricultural land increased by 74 per cent between 1997 and 2001. This growth makes organics the fastest growing segment of US agriculture. Farmers in forty-nine US states dedicated 2.2 million acres (890,688.3 hectares) of cropland and pasture to organic production systems in 2003. During the past decade sales of US organic products have grown 20 per cent or more annually. Organic food and beverage sales are estimated to have topped $15 billion in 2004, up from $3.5 billion in 1997. Sales are projected to more than double in the next three to four years or sooner with giant stores like Wal-Mart entering the organic market in a big way from 2006 onwards. As more individuals become concerned about the consumption of synthetic chemical and pesticide-laden foods, predictions are that the demand for organic produce will continue its rapid growth.

Japan now ranks as the largest Asian market for organic products. Demand for organics in other Asian countries is also growing. According to 2006 statistics, of the 6.9 million acres (2.8 million hectares) of organically managed farm land in Asia, 5.7 million acres (2.3 million hectares) are in China. China has established itself as a global producer of key organic ingredients, including soybeans, seeds and grains. The US exports an estimated 40 to 60 million dollars worth of organic goods to Japan each year and the number increases each year. Japan is also the largest importer of organic produce by weight from Australia. The Japanese people are demanding consumers who expect quality and safety in their food supply. They are also keenly aware of environmental concerns. Therefore, their demand for organic foods is expected to rise consistently.

Marketing advertisements produced by the agrochemical industry are directed toward convincing the public that chemical farming is necessary in order to feed the world's burgeoning population. However, history demonstrates how the Asian people have fed large populations for thousands of years using natural organic fertilizers.

Human and animal waste has been used for centuries as an organic fertilizer in China, Korea and Japan to grow food and maintain highly productive soils. Chemical fertilizers, employed extensively in modern Western agriculture, were not available to all countries until recent years. Asian populations have spread raw human excrement or night soil on gardens and fields for thousands of years. However, this practice was never accepted in the Western world. The use of raw night soil produces offensive odours and provides a route of transmission for various pathogenic micro-organisms, especially parasites.

Today, modern hydroponic techniques make safe the use of human and animal waste as an organic fertilizer. Using hydroponics, crops can grow without exposing individuals to untreated waste. NASA researchers successfully grew food crops while treating wastewater. See the sixth chapter for more on this subject.

As Asian countries, particularly Japan, have become highly modernized and industrialized, the practice of applying raw night soil to gardens and fields is disappearing among younger generations. The use of synthetic fertilizers in China has risen more than 600 per cent between the mid-1960s and the mid-1980s. Along with the increased use of synthetic fertilizers and discarding of sewage into rivers and streams, water pollution in China and other Asian countries is beginning to surpass water pollution levels equal to those in the US and other Western countries.

With Asian countries abandoning their centuries-old practice of applying human excreta back to the soil for food production, a crisis in environmental pollution and food shortages could emerge in the near future. With the world population at over six billion and growing, bio-technologies must be developed rapidly to utilize human and animal excreta as sources of nutrients to produce food and other plant materials for industrial uses.

Plant-based Foods for a Healthy Diet

Modern science confirms that the healthiest foods we humans can eat are the same as those eaten by our earlier ancestors. Plant-based foods such as beans, peas, lentils, whole grains, dark green leafy vegetables, nuts and fruits made up the bulk of our ancestors' diet with meat as only an occasional addition (see Fig. 4.14).

Many eat diets that are determined by a number of factors, including nationality or region, ethnicity, religious beliefs, socio-economic standing or simply cost and availability. Yet, the basics for a healthy diet remain constant. A variety of fresh, non-processed foods will generally assure that nutritional needs are met. Diet plays a significant role in longevity.

Common sense tells us that one of the best ways to determine how to live a long healthy life is to look at individuals who are at an advanced age of 90-100 years and observe

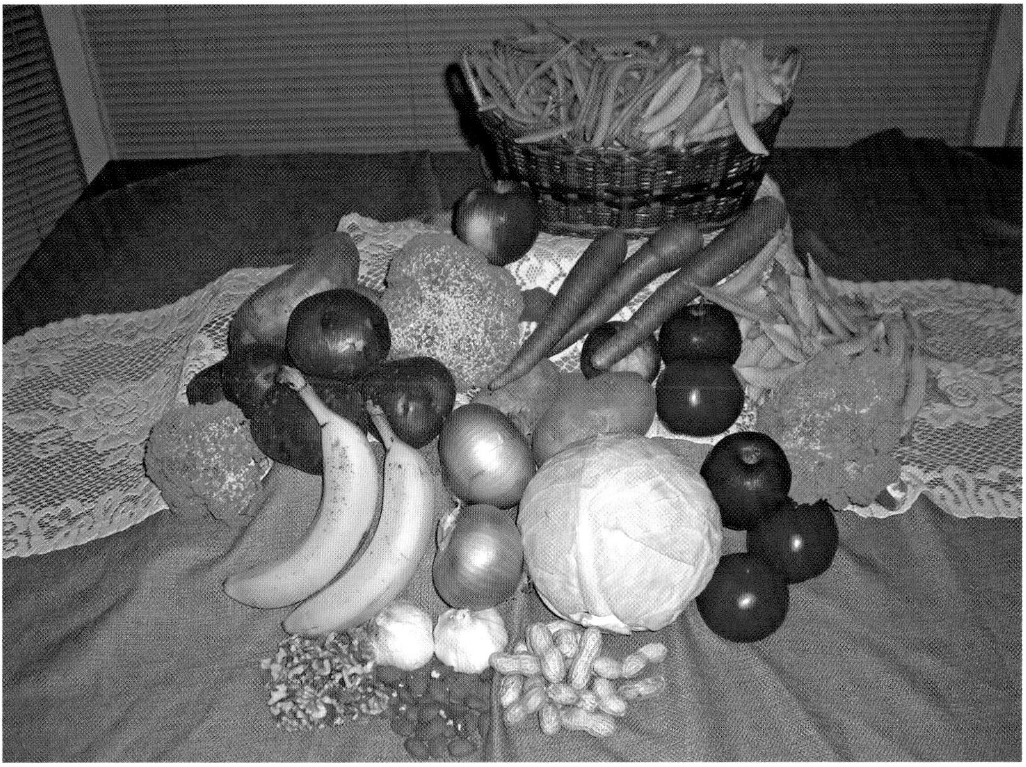

FIG. 4.14

their lifestyle and eating habits. According to a WHO study, the Japanese people have the longest, healthiest life expectancy of all people on earth. The inhabitants of Okinawa, a Japanese Prefecture (State), get 80 per cent less breast and prostate cancer and have 80 per cent fewer heart attacks than Americans. In Okinawa, there are about 34 people per one hundred thousand who are healthy at 100 years of age. In the US, only 5 to 10 individuals per one hundred thousand ever attain the age of 100.

The Okinawa Program, a book by Dr Bradley Willcox and colleagues, details a twenty-five-year study on why Okinawans generally live long, healthy lives. The answers are quite simple. Okinawans consume mostly vegetables and seafood. They drink unsweetened hot tea, not sugar-laden tea and soft drinks common in the American diet. They also get far more exercise than an average American.

There are also small pockets of people in other countries who live long, healthy lives. In Dr T.H. Ling's book, *Green Tea and Its Amazing Health Benefits*, he discusses the longevity of people who live in Ba Su, a mountainous area in the Guangxi Province of China. On 16 November 1997, the Associated Press reported that in Ba Su (population 26,000) 79 were centenarians and hundreds more were in their nineties. By contrast, in the 1990 census, only 56 of the 11 million residents of Beijing were 100 years old. In the remote Ba Su community, medical services are among the least available in China. Yet, there were almost 600 times more centenarians based upon percentage of population than in Beijing, where people have access to most, if not all, of the latest medical services and modern foods.

Individuals in Ba Su drink copious amounts of green tea and consume local fresh corn, rice and other vegetables, but eat very little meat. Their rate of heart disease is only 4.3 per cent. Juangdong Province is located just south of Guangxi Province, across from Hong Kong. This province has been highly modernized and industrialized. The people there enjoy a much higher standard of living than in other areas of China. Those living in Guangzhou, China's largest and most prosperous city in the South, have a heart disease rate of 38 per cent, nine times greater than Ba Su, only a short distance away. Therefore, the longevity of people in Ba Su cannot be attributed to modern medicine but to eating habits and lifestyle. Numerous studies have shown that children of immigrants to the US who adopt an American diet develop heart disease, cancer, diabetes, etc., at rates similar to other Americans. Therefore, genetics, in most cases, may play only a minor role in longevity.

People in Western countries generally consume the most red meat and their health and longevity suffer because of it. As early as 1961, the *Journal of the American Medical Association* (*JAMA*) stated that 90 to 97 per cent of heart disease, the cause of more than half the deaths in America, could be prevented by a vegetarian diet. People in Asian countries, on the other hand, usually have diets that are more plant-oriented, along with fish and poultry. As a result, they enjoy greater longevity, even though many have limited access to healthcare.

Many people in all cultures choose a vegetarian lifestyle, some for its health benefits and others due to religious beliefs. A 2008 *Vegetarian Times* study found that 7.3 million Americans, or 3.2 per cent of the population, are vegetarians. In the United Kingdom, a 2006 survey revealed that 6 per cent of the population, or 3.6 million, are vegetarians. These numbers rose significantly following the mad cow scare with 10 per cent claiming to eat no red meat. India has more vegetarians than the rest of the world combined, primarily driven by caste and religious beliefs. A 2006 survey found that 40 per cent of the population, or 399 million Indians, are vegetarians.

Beans, Peas and Lentils

Beans, peas and lentils are available in almost all cultures and are generally among the least expensive foods. They are very low in fat and packed with complex carbohydrates, protein and water-soluble fibre, that helps lower 'bad' cholesterol. They are also rich in folates (folic acid), vitamins, minerals, iron, potassium, calcium, magnesium and many phytonutrients.

If someone is seeking to reduce meat consumption, these are good alternative sources of protein. A variety of these vegetables should be consumed on a regular basis, at least three times a week, as an essential component of a healthy diet. They can be added to soups, salads, casseroles or simply be eaten with other vegetables, fish or meats (see Figs. 4.15 and 4.16).

CALCIUM VALUE OF BEANS

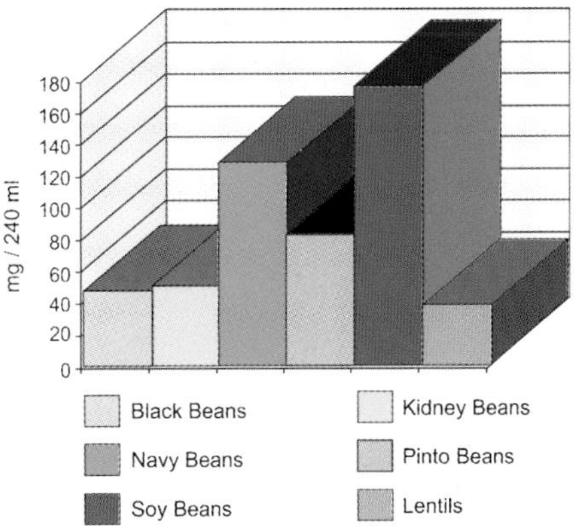

Source: USDA Nutrient Database

FIG. 4.15

PROTEIN VALUE OF BEANS

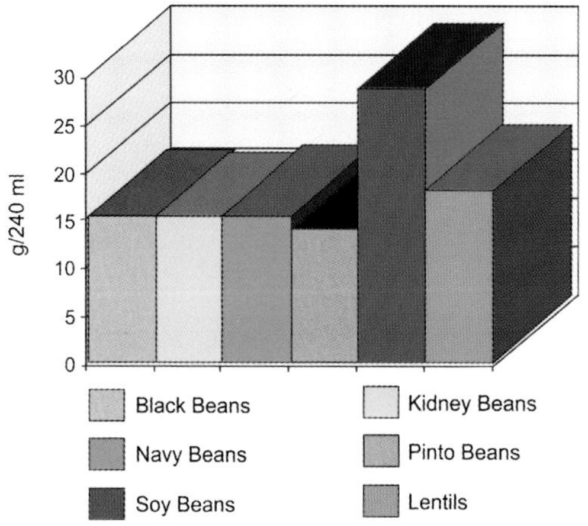

Source: USDA Nutrient Database

FIG. 4.16

Some may shy away from these nutritious foods because of their tendency to produce intestinal gas. Beans, whole grains and other vegetables with high fibre content are likely to produce this effect. Humans lack the enzyme necessary to break down these complex carbohydrates into single sugars for absorption. Instead, colon bacteria digest these starches, producing gas as a by-product. This problem can be overcome by eating smaller quantities until the digestive system becomes accustomed to them. Additionally, soaking dried beans or peas overnight in water and discarding the water will reduce some of the substances that produce gas during digestion.

Whole Grains

Grains, also called cereals, are the widely varied seeds of grasses that have been cultivated for centuries as food. Grains have been hailed as the 'staff of life' because of their historical significance for human survival. They come in all shapes, sizes and varieties including amaranth, barley, buckwheat, bulgar, corn, kamut, millet, oats, quinoa, rice, rye, sorghum, teff, wheat and wild rice.

All types of grains are good sources of complex carbohydrates, vitamins and minerals. They are naturally low in fat. Whole grains are those that have not been through a milling or refining process. The milling process removes bran and germ. As a result, refined grains have fewer nutrients and less fibre. Whole grains are better sources of fibre and other important nutrients, such as selenium, potassium and magnesium.

We have long been aware that the use of whole wheat was a more healthy choice than processed white flour. During the early 1880s, Sylvester Graham, a US Presbyterian minister, stressed the importance of eating whole-wheat flour and fresh vegetables. He became known for his now famous 'Graham crackers'. He denounced urban bakers who used refined flour. Unfortunately, he fought a losing battle. Bread made with refined flour bakes more quickly than traditional breads, producing an almost crust-less loaf. It quickly found favour with bakers and customers alike. However, its nutritional value was greatly diminished. Today, most processed foods are made with refined grains. Sadly, in industrialized nations, only about 5 per cent of grain foods that are available to consumers are in whole grain form.

Green Leafy Vegetables

Dark green leafy vegetables are important sources of many vitamins and minerals that are essential for health. They, too, are a great source of fibre and contain vitamins A, C, D, E and K, folates, iron and calcium. Research suggests that the nutrients found in dark green vegetables may prevent certain types of cancers and make the heart healthier. Some examples of green leafy vegetables are arugula, collard greens, kale, mustard greens, lettuce, spinach, turnip greens, Swiss chard, cabbage, brussel sprouts, broccoli and cauliflower.

Numerous scientific studies have shown that people who eat significant quantities of these vegetables lower their risk of disease. Certain phytochemicals found in these vegetables have been shown to have cancer-fighting properties. For example, the chemical compound, indole-3-carbinol reduces the incidence of breast and uterine cancer in women.

Nuts

A variety of nuts eaten often but in small quantities contributes to an overall healthy diet. Because of their high fat content, nuts

CALCIUM VALUE OF NUTS

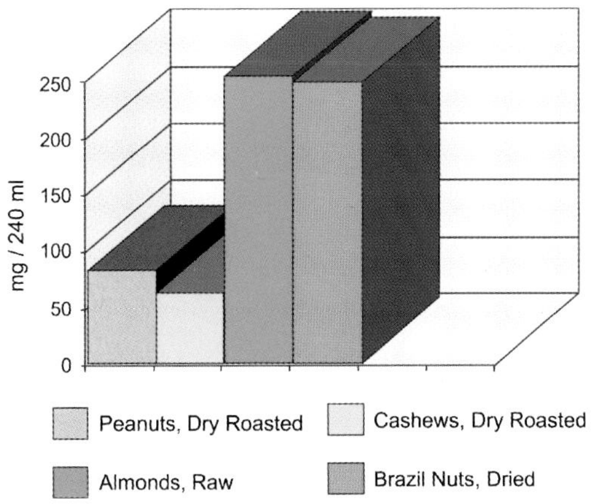

Source: USDA Nutrient Database

FIG. 4.17

PROTEIN VALUE OF NUTS

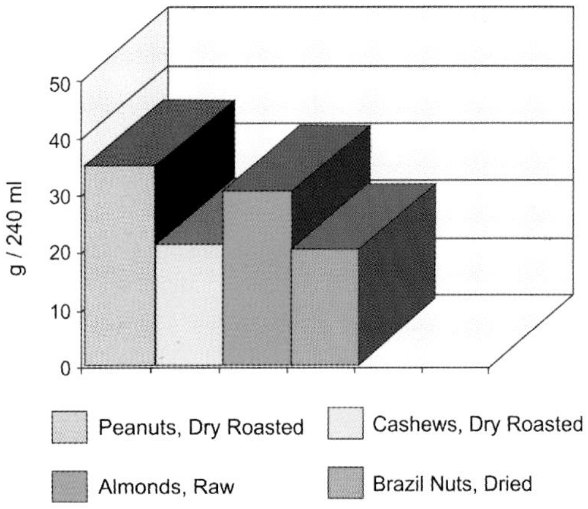

Source: USDA Nutrient Database

FIG. 4.18

have had a bad reputation for years. Although nuts are high in fat, it is mostly healthy monounsaturated oil, a more healthy form of fat. Some nuts, such as walnuts, are also excellent sources of heart-protecting omega-3 fatty acids. This 'good' fat content combined with fibre, protein, folates, magnesium, potassium, Vitamin E and Vitamin B_6 make nuts an important health food. Nuts also contain essential trace elements such as boron, zinc, copper and selenium. Recent research has proven that nuts of all kinds are full of rich flavonoids, vital nutrition and appear to give protection against some of today's most troublesome health problems (see Figs. 4.17 and 4.18).

In a large health study reported in the British Medical Journal, more than 86,000 women were observed for over twenty-three years. Data demonstrated those women who ate more than five ounces (141.5 g) of nuts per week had a significantly lower risk of heart diseases than those who ate one or less ounces (28.3 g) of nuts. The Harvard School of Public Health also conducted studies involving people who had already suffered heart attacks to see how eating nuts affected their risk of another attack. Those who ate nuts at least twice a week had a 25 per cent reduction in their risk of another heart attack, as compared to those who did not eat any nuts. For those having high blood pressure, it is important to eat unsalted or lightly salted nuts.

Scientists at the US Department of Agriculture have found that peanuts contain the heart-healthy compound, resveratrol. The findings on resveratrol in peanuts appear to support the epidemiological studies at the Harvard School of Public Health and other studies cited above. Resveratrol is also found in blueberries, cranberries, grape juice and wine. However, much more publicity has been given to its content in red wine.

These findings correspond to teachings recorded in ancient history. Viniculture (the cultivation of grapes) began thousands of years ago and was common to many cultures, including the Egyptian, Iranian, Israelite and Greek. Many religions use wine in their religious ceremonies or rituals. Its use is also recorded in ancient religious texts, such as the Bible. However, the Bible cautions against excessive intake stating that 'a little wine is good for the stomach'.

Resveratrol is not found in the pulp but in the skin of grapes, thus red wine contains more resveratrol because it is fermented longer with the skin than white wine. It is also found in non-fermented grape juice but at much lower concentrations. On an equal basis, peanuts have about half the amount of resveratrol as found in red wine.

Resveratrol has been shown to have some cancer-fighting properties as well. Research conducted at the University of Illinois at Chicago using resveratrol extracts from grapes showed a reduced risk of cancer in animals by stopping the growth of damaged cells in the body. An overall healthy diet should include some source of resveratrol.

Fruits

Fruits are a dietary staple with hundreds of varieties grown around the world. Whether wild or cultivated, some forms of fruits thrive in nearly all temperate zones. By far though, the majority grow in tropical and sub-tropical zones. Fruits are a great source of vitamins and natural sugars and their nutritional value is widely recognized today. Many of the citrus fruits originated in Southeast Asia but are now grown all around the world.

Scientific proof of the importance of citrus fruits came in 1756, when John Lind, a surgeon in the English navy, found that the scurvy common among sailors at the time could be prevented by eating oranges and lemons. Most fruits are high in vitamins A and C. Fruits are also an excellent source of minerals such as potassium, phosphorus and magnesium. With rapid shipping methods throughout the world, a wide variety of fruits are readily available in today's markets. These should form part of one's staple diet.

Other Plants

Other plants are beneficial to the human diet but are added predominantly as flavour enhancers and spices. Onions and garlic are both rich in powerful compounds containing sulphur, which is primarily responsible for their pungent odours and for many of their health-promoting properties. Onions are very rich in chromium, a trace mineral that helps cells respond to insulin, plus Vitamin C and numerous flavonoids. The regular consumption of onions and garlic has been shown to lower high cholesterol levels and high blood pressure and both help prevent diabetes and heart disease. Onions also significantly reduce the risk of developing colon cancer.

A wide variety of spices has been used for centuries to add flavour to an otherwise bland diet and as preservatives. Many plants serve as a source of fresh flavour-enhancers and are commonly grown on kitchen windowsills or in backyard herb gardens. More often than not, they are dried and ground into powder and sold in the market. The kinds and quantities of spices used in culinary dishes are as varied as the many cultures from which they are derived. It is safe to assume that the wide array of spices does not only add flavour to foods but goes a long way toward insuring overall health and vitality.

SUMMARY

Almost everyone has access to gardens. In urban environments, gardens are most typically found in public venues, parks, etc. In suburban areas, most homes display some form of exterior landscaping. Many enthusiastically provide ornamental flowering gardens, fruit trees and vegetable gardens to not only provide a beautiful, aesthetic setting for their home but to also provide fresh, healthy fruits and vegetables for their family. The uniqueness of each garden makes it a place of refuge for the inhabitants whose personality is often reflected within the landscaping. As one travels to more rural areas, the landscape often turns to agricultural lands dedicated to feeding the world's burgeoning population.

Regardless of the size of one's garden, it is incumbent that the owner show environmental responsibility. As we race to eradicate weeds and insects, grow greener grass, produce bigger and better flowers and vegetables, we should be mindful of the use of harsh, synthetic chemicals. One of the leading sources of pollution in urban areas is the runoff of chemicals from home landscaping. Keep in mind that whatever enters our storm drains will eventually find its way into our rivers and streams. Agricultural runoff is an even bigger environmental problem and has led to outbreaks of diseases in some areas.

The introduction of innovative new concepts that view gardens as mini-ecosystems where natural processes balance and recycle our waste products is an exciting new era in landscaping. These ideas may prove vital in helping to maintain a healthy environment and lend an excitement to gardening in the twenty-first century.

Medicinal Plants

Since the beginning of civilization people have used plants as medicine. Throughout history people have held the belief that plants possess healing powers. Many prescribed medications would not exist without plants. In the US, approximately 25 per cent of prescription medicines contain plant-derived chemicals, while many other medicines are made from synthetic chemicals. Until the late nineteenth century, physicians treated most diseases with herbal medicines. The great abbeys of England and France maintained gardens with medicinal plants and they often exchanged plants with one another. In fact, these medicinal gardens were often located next to infirmaries. In many countries today, herbal medicines continue as the preferred treatment method. The WHO estimates that up to 80 per cent of the world's population still relies mainly on herbal medicine for primary healthcare, especially in developing nations and rainforest countries.

In the Western Pacific region, a well-established medical system exists, based upon Chinese medical classics, which utilizes acupuncture and herbal therapy, principally with complex combinations of herbs. Traditional medicine that originated in China has been adapted to local conditions and needs in countries such as Vietnam, Malaysia, Singapore, Korea and Japan.

India is second only to China in the production of medicinal herbs. Medicinal use of plants in India dates back thousands of years. The science is known as Ayurveda (*ayu* means life, and *veda* means knowledge). Thus, this science is known as the knowledge of life. More than 2,500 species have been identified for medicinal purposes, making India recognized worldwide for its contributions to herbal medicine.

Japanese herbal medicine or Kampo is part of traditional East Asian medicine. Kampo is fundamentally a clinical system based upon the classical medical literature dating back to the Han Dynasty in ancient China. In Japan today, 75 per cent of physicians use at least some traditional Kampo formulas. These formulas are available in most pharmacies by prescription or under the advice of specially trained pharmacists and differ significantly from Western-style herbology. In Western countries, herbology uses only individual herbs or their standardized extraction. Kampo mixes together multiple raw herbs according to specific ancient formulas and then performs an extraction on the entire mixture. Since its establishment in 1950, the Japan Society for Oriental Medicine has played an important role in helping Kampo medicine achieve its high status in current Japanese healthcare.

Chinese herbalists discovered many medicinal plants, notably ginseng, tea, sesame, garlic and cinnamon. In 1590, Li Shih-chen published his landmark fifty-two-volume *Pen Tsao Kang Mu* (the catalogue of medicinal herbs). He included 1,094 medicinal plants. Today, Chinese medicine employs about 300 herbs, 150 of which are considered indispensable. These include Chinese angelica (dang gui), burdock, chrysanthemum, cinnamon, dandelion, garlic, gentian, ginger, ginseng, hawthorn, liquorice, lotus, mint, rhubarb, skullcap, senna and tea.

Starting in the mid-nineteenth century, European colonists introduced Western medicine in China. Today, Western and Chinese medicines are integrated and Western-trained physicians practise alongside traditional herbalists and acupuncturists. Many Chinese physicians also practise in Western countries using traditional Chinese medicine. A turning point in American acceptance of Chinese medicine occurred in 1972 when President Richard Nixon first visited China.

Development of the synthetic chemical industry in the early twentieth century brought about a dramatic change in Western medicine. By the late twentieth century, most herbal medicines in the US had been replaced with synthetic chemicals. However, recent concerns about the harmful side effects of prescription medicines have led to an explosive growth in the nutritional supplement market and herbal medicines are making a dramatic comeback.

An article published in the April 1998 issue of *JAMA* indicated that as many as 137,000 Americans die each year from adverse reactions to properly prescribed medications and as many as 2.2 million are seriously injured. Another article published in the January 2000 issue of *JAMA* indicated that the third leading cause of death in America today is attributed to the medical industry. Due to the toxic side effects of many synthetic prescription medications, a growing number of physicians practising 'traditional' medicine are also prescribing less toxic herbal medicines.

Herbal medicines generally take longer to produce beneficial effects than synthetic prescription drugs. However, they exhibit far fewer side effects. Today's modern methods for extracting and concentrating the active compounds from herbs now produce stronger, more effective herbal medicines. But care should be exercised with both prescription and herbal medicines, especially when taken in combination. Always consult a healthcare provider for possible interactions.

Vitamins, minerals and herbs are recognized in the US as dietary supplements and for their role in promoting health. But herbal products do not fall under the controlling authority of the US Food and Drug Administration (FDA). Therefore, it is legal to market herbal products as either food or dietary supplements, even though they may actually be medicines. The dietary supplement market and the vitamin and herbal medicine industry have grown so fast in the US during recent years that there is a shortage of trained doctors with the expertise to steer patients to the use of only highly purified and standardized herbal extracts. In the US and many other countries, herbal medicines lack strict quality control. Unfortunately, many unscrupulous individuals have been attracted to this multi-billion dollar industry and have been abusing customers through the sale of non-standardized products. In 2001, the *Nutrition Business Journal* estimated the total sales of dietary supplements at 17.8 billion dollars.

SOME OF THE MORE IMPORTANT MEDICINAL PLANTS

CINNAMON (*Cinnamomum zeylanicum*) or CHINESE CINNAMON (*Cinnamomum cassia*)

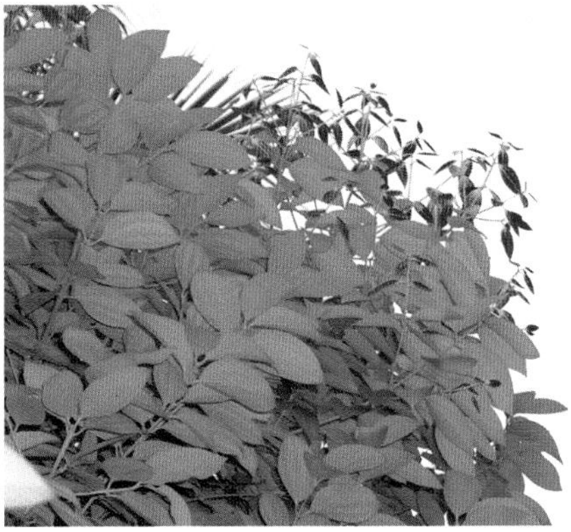

Ancient Chinese herbalists used cinnamon as a treatment for fever, diarrhoea and menstrual problems. The biblical Hebrews, Greeks and Romans adapted cinnamon as a spice, perfume and treatment for indigestion. By the seventeenth century, Europeans considered cinnamon primarily a kitchen spice. In healing, they used it only to mask the bitterness of other herbs.

During the nineteenth century, cinnamon was used for stomach cramps, nausea, and diarrhoea and infant colic. Japanese researchers report that cinnamon helps reduce blood pressure. In Germany, cinnamon is approved for indigestion, abdominal distress, bloating and flatulence. Like other culinary spices, it has antiseptic properties. It kills many pathogenic bacteria, fungi and viruses.

Research published in the *Diabetes Care Journal* demonstrated the ability of 1, 3 and 6 grammes of cinnamon in reducing fasting glucose levels from 18 to 29 per cent. It also reduced triglycerides from 23 to 30 per cent, LDL cholesterol from 7 to 27 per cent and total cholesterol from 12 to 26 per cent.

Cinnamon is not grown in the US. Most of the supply comes from Asia and the West Indies. The trees reach a height of 10 m. Collectors strip the aromatic bark from young branches no more than three years old. The bark of *Cinnamomum zeylanicum* is generally considered to be of better quality than bark from *Cinnamomum cassia*.

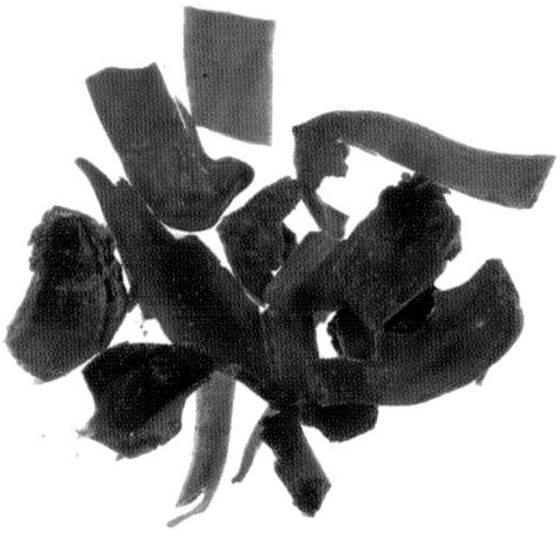

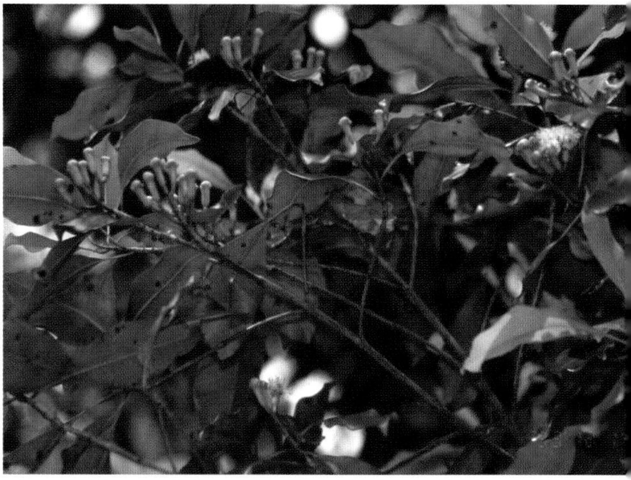

CLOVE (*Eugenia caryophyllata* or *Syzygium aromaticum*)

Clove comes from the aromatic dried flower buds of a tree in the family *Myrtaceae*. It is native to Indonesia and is used as a spice in cuisines all over the world. Cloves are harvested primarily in Zanzibar, Indonesia and Madagascar; they are also grown in India, Sri Lanka, Brazil and the West Indies. Cloves are an important incense material in Chinese and Japanese culture. The oil of cloves is widely used in aromatherapy and to treat toothaches. The compound responsible for the clove's aroma is eugenol. It is the main component of the essential oil extracted from clove, and is present from 72 to 90 per cent. Eugenol has pronounced antiseptic and anaesthetic properties.

FLAX (*Linum usitatissimum*)

Flax is one of the most ancient cultivated plants and is grown for its seeds and fibres. It is most widely known for the fibre obtained from its stems. The plant was grown and used by early Egyptians and Greeks to make linen cloth. Flax fibres were found in burial chambers that date back to 3000 BC. The oil from flaxseeds is known as linseed oil. It is used widely in paints and varnishes.

Flax has a long history of use in herbal medicine. In China and India, flax is recommended for treatment in a variety of ailments, including constipation, cough, urinary problems and skin irritations. In India, flax is known regionally as *akshi*, *jawas* or *alsi*. It is a key ingredient in chutneys.

Only in the past few years have Americans begun to view flaxseeds as 'health food'.

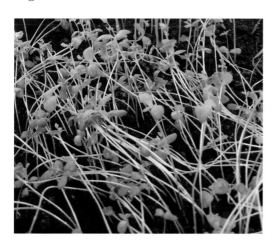

Flaxseeds are a rich source of compounds called lignans. Lignans can have strong antioxidant properties that can help block the damaging effects of free radicals that primarily accelerate cancer and heart-related diseases. Most of the lignans found in flaxseeds are in the meal, which is the non-oil part of the seed. Flaxseeds are also rich in omega-3 fatty acids and are very high in fibre. Because of all these three components, flaxseeds have become one of the most promising health food products.

Some of the same chemical compounds in flaxseeds that help fight cancer also show promise for reducing the risk of heart disease. Studies have shown that the omega-3 fatty acids appear to reduce the incidence of blood clotting that can increase the risk of stroke and heart disease.

Because flaxseeds have a hard protective shell, they should be ground before use. An easy way to produce fine-ground flaxseed is by using a spice or coffee grinder. The ground meal can then be added to cereals, oatmeal or to muffins, bread and other baked goods. Flaxseed meal has a slightly sweet, nutty taste. The oils in flaxseeds spoil rapidly in warm temperatures. Therefore, flaxseed oil or freshly ground flaxseed requires refrigeration for safe storage.

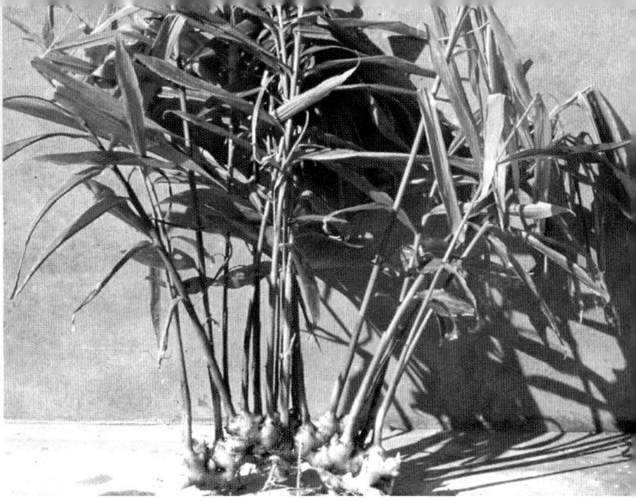

GINGER (*Zingiber officinale*)

Ginger figured prominently in early Chinese herbal medicine. It was recommended for colds, fever, chills, tetanus and leprosy. Chinese physicians also prescribed ginger to treat arthritis, ulcers and kidney problems.

Ancient Greek traders learned of the Asian practice of using ginger as a nausea-preventing digestive aid. They took the herb with them on their journey back to Greece. After big meals, it was wrapped in sweetened bread and eaten as a stomach settler. Eventually, the Greeks began baking the herb into the sweet bread, which later evolved into cookies and gingerbread.

In England and her American colonies, ginger was incorporated into a stomach-soothing drink called ginger beer, the forerunner of today's ginger ale. Ginger ale is still a popular home remedy for diarrhoea, nausea and vomiting.

Ginger's anti-nausea action first received scientific validation in 1982 in a study conducted by researchers at Brigham Young University (USA) and published in the British medical journal, the *Lancet*. Since that study, Swedish, Danish and Italian researchers have confirmed ginger's value for the prevention of motion and morning sickness. Many modern studies have confirmed what the Chinese herbalists reported centuries ago on the medical value of ginger.

Fresh ginger is also used extensively in Japanese and Asian cooking as flavouring. It is considered to be one of the most important and indispensable spices in Indian culinary practices and is used in both vegetarian and meat-based dishes. In Japan, its slices are routinely served between courses of sushi to clear the palate and aid in digestion. Ginger tea is a good herbal tonic for influenza (flu) because of its soothing qualities and its antiviral abilities; and it is widely used in India to cure sore throats.

Ginger is grown in many parts of the world. It is a tropical perennial that grows from a tuberous underground stem or rhizome. Each year, the plant produces a round, one-metre stem with thin, pointed, lance-shaped 25 cm leaves and a single, large yellow-and-purple flower. Ginger is also grown indoors in deep containers. When grown indoors, it needs warmth, plenty of water and high humidity that is best found in greenhouse environments.

GINKGO / MAIDENHAIR TREE (*Ginkgo biloba*)

The ginkgo tree is the longest surviving tree species on the planet, dating back millions of years. Ginkgo can be found planted in many cities throughout the world because it is a hardy shade tree that is resistant to air pollution, insects and diseases and can live to be 1,000 years old. The ginkgo has brilliant green leaves that are fan-shaped with parallel veins with a notch in the middle that divides the leaf into two lobes giving it the name 'biloba'. The Chinese have used ginkgo nuts for thousands of years as medicine for many ailments.

One of the most popular usages of ginkgo leaf extracts is for increasing circulation to the brain, supplying oxygen that can help improve mental clarity. This herb also helps in the prevention and treatment of circulatory problems. Like aspirin, it acts as a mild anticoagulant by inhibiting the aggregation of blood platelets and may be helpful in preventing strokes. This herb contains strong antioxidants that may help stop the damage to organs from free radicals. It, like aspirin, also has anti-inflammatory properties.

Standardized leaf extracts contain ginkgo flavonglycosides (bioflavonoids) and terpene lactones as its active parts. When purchasing *ginkgo biloba* capsules, make sure the standardized extract contains 24 per cent ginkgo flavonglycosides and 6 per cent terpene lactones. *Ginkgo biloba* should not be taken by anyone on blood thinners or daily aspirin without consulting their physician.

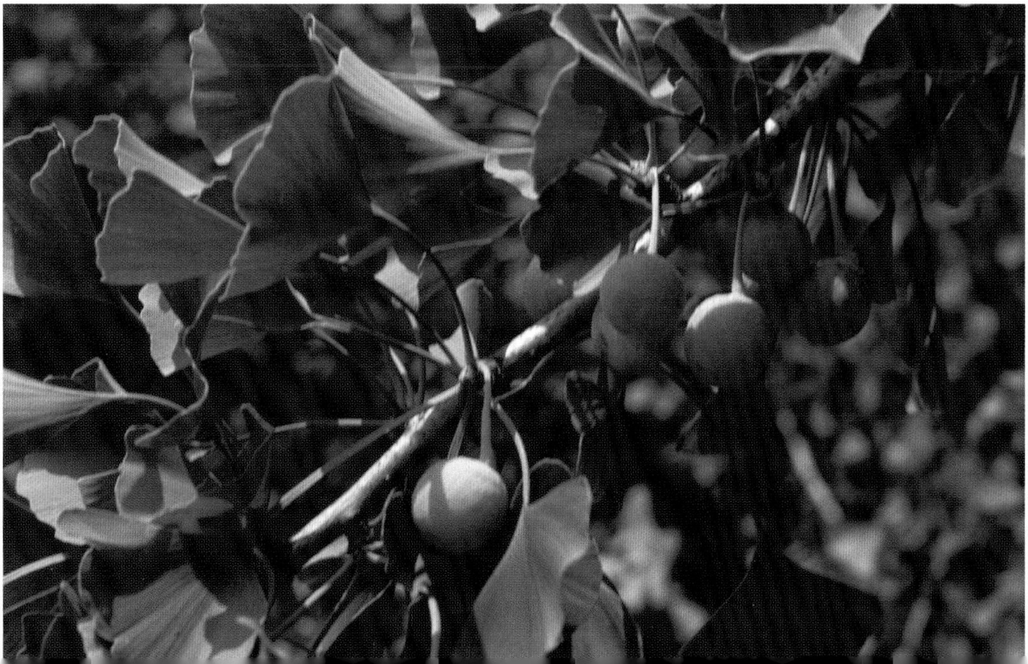

GINSENG – CHINESE / KOREAN / JAPANESE (*Panax ginseng*) or AMERICAN (*Panax quinquefolius*)

Ginseng has a fleshy, multi-branched root. The ancient Chinese called the plant 'man root' or *jen shen*, which eventually entered the English language as *jinseng*. Unlike other Asian herbs that became favourites in the West, ginseng remained relatively unknown in Europe until the eighteenth century. By the 1770s, ginseng became popular in America. The search for ginseng played an important role in the exploration of western Pennsylvania, West Virginia, Kentucky and Tennessee.

For centuries, Chinese healers have prescribed ginseng to normalize blood pressure, improve blood circulation and prevent heart disease. Ginseng is believed to increase estrogen levels in women and has been suggested as an aphrodisiac. The primary active ingredients in ginseng are compounds collectively known as ginsenosides. However, ginseng is difficult to grow.

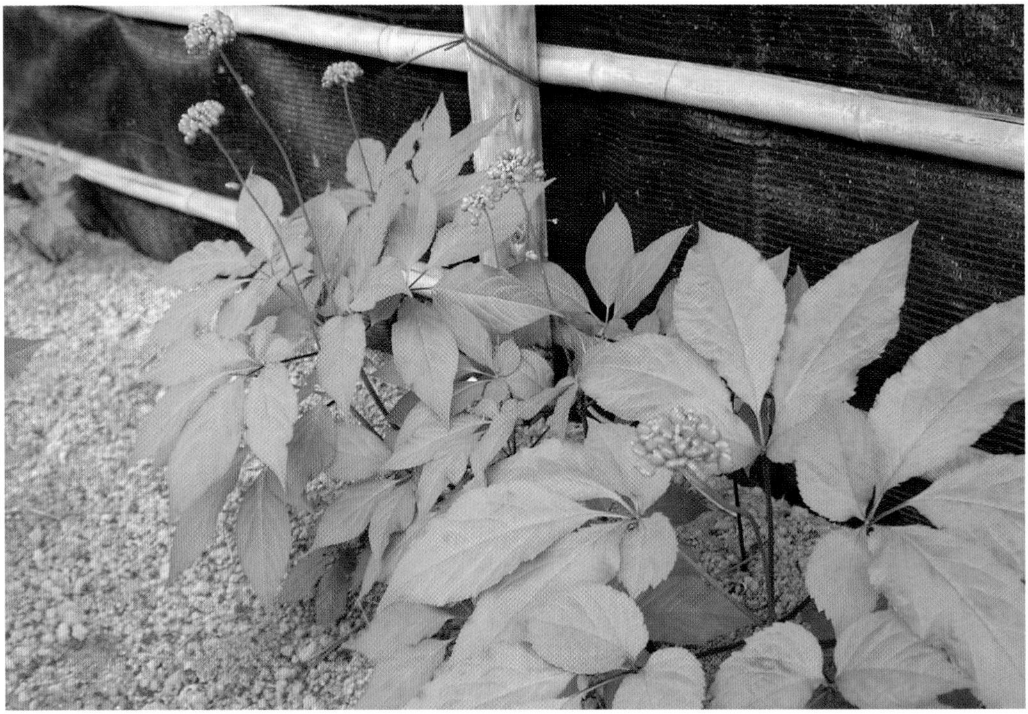

TEA (*Camellia sinensis*)

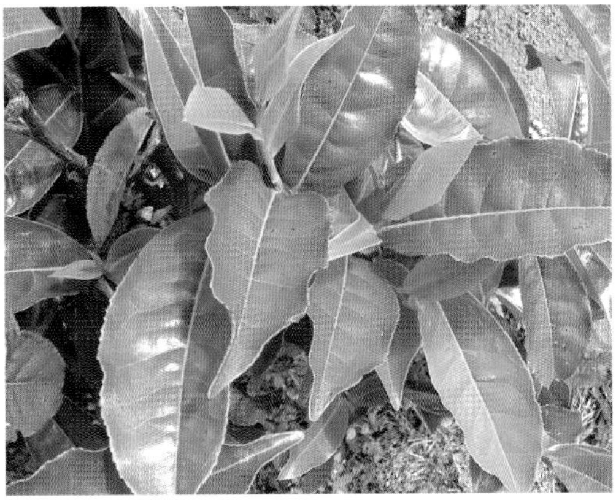

Tea is second to only water as the most popular beverage worldwide. There are three types of tea: green, black and oolong. All are produced from the leaves of *Camellia sinensis* but vary in their extraction process. Green tea, preferred in East Asian countries, is made from leaves that are simply dried and crumbled. Black tea, preferred in most South Asian and Western countries, is made when the leaves are first dried and then fermented. Oolong tea is partially fermented.

For thousands of years, the Chinese people have enjoyed green tea. According to Dr Tiong-Hung Ling, author of *Green Tea and Its Amazing Health Benefits*, the oldest written record of tea in Chinese history is the Hua Yang National Record (206 BC). Tea was first used as a herb before it became a common drink. Japanese monks who went to China to learn Buddhism were the first to introduce tea to Japan. Planting of tea in Japan began in AD 805.

The Dutch East India Company introduced tea in Holland in 1610. By 1640, its popularity had spread to England. The British upper class practised the '4 o'clock tea time' that remains popular till today. The demand for tea encouraged England to colonize India, Sri Lanka (formerly Ceylon) and Hong Kong. In 1773, the British levied a tax on all tea sold in the North American colonies. A tax revolt incited by the famous cry 'no taxation without representation' led to the Boston Tea Party where angry colonialists dumped shiploads of tea into the harbour, helping to trigger the American Revolutionary War.

While tea has been used in Chinese medicine for at least 3,000 years, only in recent years have scientists identified the chemical components of tea. The health benefits from drinking tea, especially green tea, are now a well-established fact. Green tea is produced from leaves that are steamed to soften them, then rolled and dried. Black tea is made by withering the leaves by air or heat, and then broken so that oxygen reacts with enzymes in the leaves. This generates a fermentation process that darkens the tea.

In the early 1980s, Japanese scientists discovered that tea contains the powerful antioxidant compounds known as polyphenols. These compounds help prevent and repair cell damage that lead to heart disease, most cancers and many other degenerative diseases. Some of the antioxidants in green tea are twenty-five times as powerful as Vitamin E, which is known to reduce the risk of heart attack. Because of the mild processing techniques used to produce green tea, most of the polyphenols remain intact.

The polyphenols called catechins appear to be most important in providing cancer protection. A 1994 study published in the *Journal of the National Cancer Institute* indicated that green tea drinkers in Shanghai cut their risk of oesophageal cancer by 57 to 60 per cent. It is also interesting to note that although Japanese green tea drinkers have a higher rate of smoking, they also have a lower rate of lung cancer than Americans. This is most likely attributable to their diet and high consumption rate of green tea. The fermentation process that converts green tea into black tea eliminates 85 per cent of the catechins. Therefore, green tea is much healthier than black tea.

Green tea has also been shown to reduce the risk of several other cancers, including colorectal, pancreatic, lung and breast cancers. Stimulants in tea also help to open bronchial passages and the astringent tannins in tea help ease diarrhoea.

HAWTHORN (*Crataegus cuneata*)

John Wesley, an eighteenth-century English clergyman and founder of the Methodist church, accidentally discovered the healing power of the hawthorn berry. Wesley observed that when his horses became exhausted they would nibble on hawthorn berries and recover quickly. He began to offer members of his church hawthorn berries as an energy tonic and saw excellent results. At the end of the nineteenth century, hawthorn was popularized by an Irish doctor who used it to treat patients with congestive heart failure.

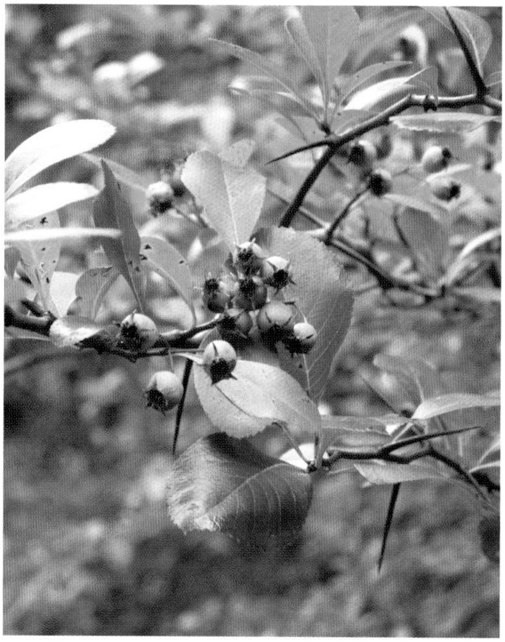

Today we know that hawthorn acts on the body in two ways. It dilates the blood vessels, especially the coronary vessels, reducing peripheral resistance (the force against blood flow) and thus lowering the blood pressure. It also dilates blood vessels in other parts of the body allowing blood to circulate more freely and thus reducing strain on the heart.

Hawthorn's action is not immediate but develops very slowly. Its toxicity is low, causing problems only when taken in large doses. For high blood pressure, some doctors recommend taking 100 to 300 mg of a standardized hawthorn extract three times a day. Nutritionally oriented doctors commonly use extracts of the leaves and flowers. Standardized extracts contain 2.2 per cent flavonoids. If traditional berry preparations are used, the recommendation is at least 4 to 5 grammes per day. For the treatment of heart disease, other doctors recommend taking 80 mg twice a day.

HORSERADISH (*Amoracia rusticana or Armoraca lapathifolia*)

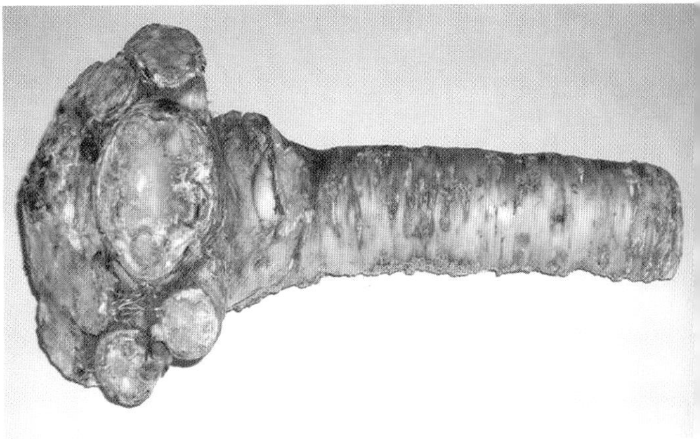

The earliest account of horseradish comes from thirteenth century Western Europe where Germans and Danes used it as a condiment, stimulant and digestive medicine. It was introduced into England in the sixteenth century where it was used to treat hoarseness and coughs. It was brought to the United States in the nineteenth century.

Horseradish continues to climb up the condiment ladder with commercial cultivation launched by German immigrants into the Midwest in America. Sixty per cent of all horseradish produced in the US is grown in Illinois, where it is an important crop. Most of the crop is crushed and mixed into relishes and sauces. It is also commonly used to add a spicy taste to roast beef, fish and oysters. It is consumed in India in spiced vegetables and in salads.

A new study from the University of Illinois shows that horseradish has substantial quantities of glucosinolates, compounds that have been shown to increase human resistance to cancer. Glucosinolates increase the liver's ability to detoxify carcinogens and may suppress the growth of existing cancerous tumours according to Dr Mosbah Kushad, associate professor of Food Crop Systems at the University of Illinois. This research was published in October 2004 in the *Journal of Agriculture and Food Chemistry*. English scientists also found that horseradish could destroy cancer cells. Horseradish differs from wasabi in that it has a white root, whereas wasabi has a green root. Wasabi is more expensive and difficult to grow. Most wasabi is grown in Japan and exported around the world.

High intake of horseradish may suppress the thyroid hormone causing low thyroid activity. Therefore, excessive consumption of horseradish is not recommended.

LAVENDER (*Lavandula angustifolia*)

For thousands of years lavender has been used as a digestive aid, sleeping aid and tranquilizer for people who are anxious, restless or emotionally troubled. Because of its mood-altering effects, lavender is also considered an antidepressant.

The essential oil extracted from lavender flowers is chemically very complex, containing more than 150 compounds. When rubbed on the skin, the oil penetrates rapidly and can be detected in the blood in five minutes. To prepare an infusion, use 5 to 15 ml of lavender flowers per 250 ml of boiling water. Steep for ten minutes and strain. Drink up to 750 ml per day.

For an aromatherapy massage, apply a few drops of lavender oil directly to the skin or blend it into a commercial massage lotion (ten drops of oil per ounce 28 ml of lotion).

Native to the Mediterranean, lavender is a pleasantly aromatic, woody, branching perennial shrub that grows to about one metre. Its narrow, fuzzy leaves change colour from grey to green as they mature. In summer, lavender produces small blue or purple flowers that develop in clusters on spikes 13 to 20 cm long. There are many species of lavender. All prefer sunny locations for growth.

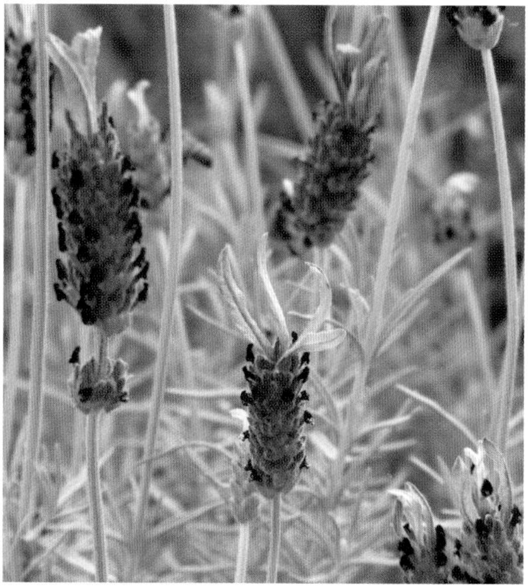

MILK THISTLE (*Silybum marianum*)

Milk thistle is native to Kashmir in the Indian subcontinent. It is a weedy plant that can be grown in temperate climates throughout the world. It normally reaches 2 to 3 m in height and produces large, prickly leaves. When broken, the leaves and stems produce milky sap from which the plant derives its name. This plant produces reddish purple flowers that are surrounded with sharp needles.

Milk thistle has been used as a liver tonic for more than 2,000 years. In 1968, German scientists identified three liver-protecting compounds in milk thistle seeds. In combination, these chemical compounds are called silymarin. Commission E is the expert panel that evaluates herbal medicine for the German government and is the equivalent of the US Food and Drug Administration. The Commission approves milk thistle extract as a treatment for liver conditions.

Many European studies of silymarin have demonstrated its value in treating patients with liver problems associated with hepatitis, mushroom poisoning, cirrhosis of the liver and drug-induced liver damage. Silymarin is a powerful antioxidant that induces the repair of damaged liver cells while stimulating the immune system. The recommended dosage of a standardized extract is one capsule containing 70 to 210 mg of silymarin three times a day.

PARSLEY (*Petroselinum crispum*)

Parsley was not widely used in ancient medicine, mainly due to folklore in various cultures having portrayed it negatively. Roman physicians prescribed parsley as a mild diuretic. They also chewed sprigs to freshen their breath. It is this practice that led to the garnishing of parsley on plates served in restaurants today. Unfortunately, most parsley arrives back at the kitchen uneaten. Parsley contains a high level of chlorophyll, an active ingredient in many breath fresheners on the market today.

Parsley is a rich source of calcium, iron and vitamins A and C. It also contains natural antispasmodic properties that aid in digestion. Many recommend steeping parsley leaves in

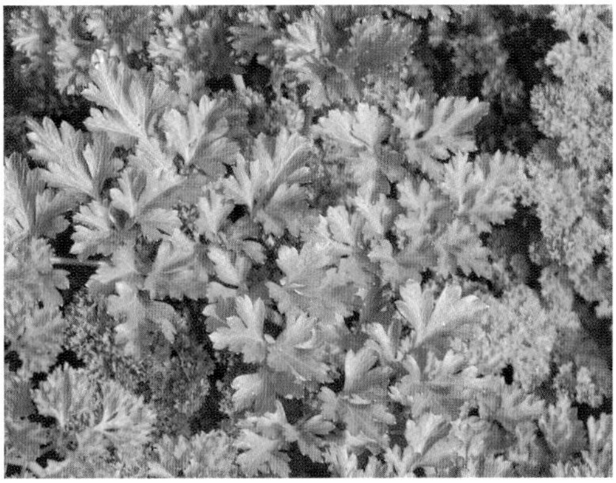

hot water for several minutes to make a weak tea. Then, sip the tea slowly following a meal. For a pleasant tasting infusion, use 10 ml of dried leaves or roots or 5 ml of crushed seeds per 250 ml of boiling water. Steep for ten minutes, then strain. Drink up to 750 ml a day. However, this dosage is not recommended if you are pregnant, nursing or taking prescription diuretics.

Parsley is a small herb that reaches 30 cm the first year and up to one metre the following year. It is a biannual but should be cultivated as an annual. The top is the portion of plant commonly used as a garnish. It is bright green with feathery, deeply divided leaves. Depending upon the variety, the leaves may be curly or flat. In the second year, it may produce tiny yellow-green flowers that develop on an umbrella-like canopy.

Coriander (British) or cilantro (US), whose botanical name is *Coriander sativum*, bears a resemblance to its relative Italian leaf, parsley. It has similar culinary and medicinal properties as parsley.

ROSEMARY (*Rosmarinus officinalis*)

Rosemary is a traditional herb commonly grown in backyard herb gardens and is a favourite in various meat dishes. Its use dates back to ancient times. Rosemary has strong antibacterial and antifungal properties. It is these qualities that led the ancients to preserve meats by wrapping them in crushed rosemary leaves. It also imparted a pleasing, aromatic flavour to the meat. Meat spoils in part due to the oxidation of fats, causing it to go rancid. The oil in rosemary contains powerful antioxidants. These antioxidants act to repress micro-organisms that lead to infection. Rosemary also has antispasmodic properties. In Germany, it is approved as a treatment for indigestion.

As an aromatic culinary herb, rosemary may help relieve symptoms in the respiratory tract caused by colds, flu and allergy. For this purpose, use 5 ml of crushed rosemary per 250 ml of boiling water. Steep for ten to fifteen minutes, then strain. Drink up to 750 ml per day.

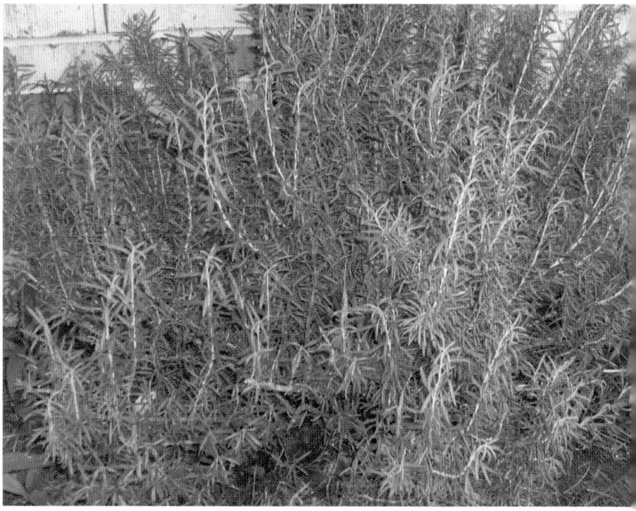

Rosemary leaves are coated with volatile aromatic oils. These oils are potent and may cause irritation to the stomach, kidney and intestinal irritation. It is best to not ingest concentrated rosemary oil. The oil is primarily used in aromatherapy.

Rosemary is an evergreen perennial shrub native to hot regions such as the Mediterranean. It prefers light, well-drained soil and full sun. It produces small, light blue flowers in summer and is fairly cold hardy. The leaves are typically stripped from the twig and rubbed onto meats, particularly lamb and poultry.

SAGE (*Salvia officinalis*)

The botanical family name *Salvia* is derived from the Latin word *salvere* which means 'to save', thus implying its importance. It is a common culinary herb, first used by Greeks and Romans as a meat preservative. Like rosemary, sage contains strong antioxidants which slow spoilage when added to food. Today, it is widely used with pork and poultry.

Dutch explorers introduced sage to the Chinese during the sixteenth century. The Chinese thought so highly of the herb that they traded the Dutch three pounds of their own tea for each pound of sage. Chinese physicians used sage to treat a variety of ailments, including gastric problems, insomnia and depression. Today, naturopaths recommend sage as an external poultice for wounds or insect bites; as a gargle for sore throat and bleeding gums and as an infusion to reduce perspiration. Studies have shown that sage can reduce perspiration by as much as 50 per cent.

Sage contains relatively high levels of a toxic chemical called thujone. In large amounts, thujone causes a variety of symptoms that can culminate in convulsions. The heat used in preparing a sage infusion destroys much of the thujone in sage. However, concentrated sage oil is toxic and should not be ingested.

Sage is a perennial evergreen shrub that may reach one metre in height. Its leaves are oval-shaped, velvety and grey-green in colour. It prefers well-drained, moderately rich soil and full sun. It generally blooms

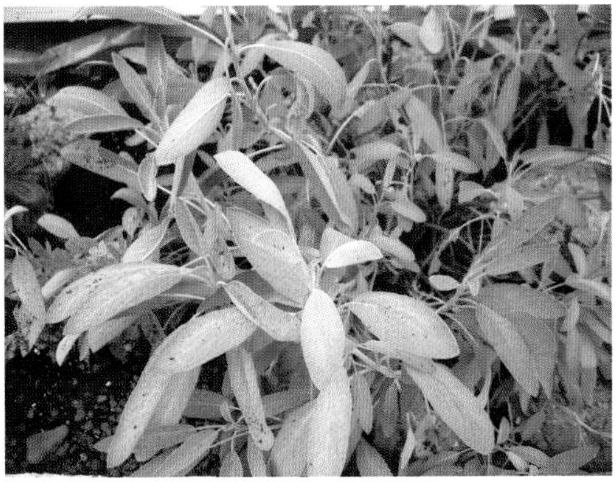

around June, producing small pink, white, blue or purple flowers. It is a cold hardy plant. It is easily preserved by drying bundled sprigs. After drying, store it in an airtight container.

SAW Palmetto (*Serenoa repens* and *S. serrulata*)

Saw palmetto is derived from the dark berries of a small south-eastern US palm tree (*Serenoa repens, S. serrulata*) with sword-like leaves that grow in a fan shape. Saw palmetto extract sales have boomed in recent years as studies have repeatedly shown that it can increase urinary flow, decrease frequency of urination and reduce discomfort associated with prostate enlargement (benign prostatic hyperplasia).

Fat-soluble saw palmetto extracts standardized to contain 85 to 95 per cent fatty acids and biologically active sterols appear to prevent the conversion of testosterone into dihydrotestosterone, which may cause excessive cell growth in the prostate. Crude berries are less expensive than the standardized, fat-soluble extracts, but will not produce similar results. The recommended dose is 160 mg of the standardized extract twice daily with meals.

Saw palmetto is sold in capsules and softgels. It is frequently combined with pygeum (*Pygeum africanum*), a herb with a somewhat less-established reputation for improving prostate health. Few side effects have been reported with saw palmetto. However, its long-term use could possibly interfere with erectile functions.

ST JOHN'S WORT (*Hypericum perforatum*)

St John's wort (also called St Johnswort) is one of the most popular of plant medicines and is referred to as 'Nature's antidepressant'. Although this plant can be an aggressive, noxious weed to some, it is a valuable medicine to others. As early as 1633, herbalists wrote of hypericum's value in treating burns. Today, St John's wort is primarily used for treating depression.

St John's wort is a perennial that grows throughout the US, Canada and Europe. The flowering tops, usually a mixture of bright yellow buds and open flowers, are the primary source of the plant's medicine. The blooms are most brilliant around the time of the feast of John the Baptist on 25 June. This is believed to be from where the plant derived its name. The petals contain black dots. When rubbed between the fingers, these dots give off a deep red colour that some claim contributes to the plant's name by representing blood from St John's beheading.

The two compounds, hypericin and hyperforin, are believed to play an important role in the plant's antidepressant effect. Most studies on the antidepressant properties of St John's wort have been conducted largely outside the US during the late 1990s. Results have been impressive and conclude that St John's wort works well for mild to moderate depression. In most of these studies, the daily dose of the extract was 300 mg three times a day.

A study conducted in Germany and published in the *British Medical Journal* (September 2000) indicated that 74 per cent of patients given 350 mg of St John's wort extract improved while only 50 per cent of the patients receiving the placebo showed any improvement. But because St John's wort extract may interact with certain prescription drugs, anyone taking any prescription medicine should check with their physician before taking this herbal medicine. Standardized extracts of St John's wort should contain 0.3 per cent hypericin, the active ingredient.

SWEET BASIL (*Ocimum basilicum*)

Basil is a popular culinary herb and its essential oils have been used extensively for many years in food production, perfumery and many other products. Herbalists have also recommended basil for stomach cramps, vomiting and constipation. Basil essential oils have exhibited anti-microbial activity against a wide range of bacteria, yeast and moulds. Although basil and its essential oils have demonstrated many health benefits, its major use is in enhancing the flavour of foods such as tomato sauce, pesto, pizza and cheese.

There are dozens of known varieties of basil, with sweet basil being the most commonly grown. Basil is native to India and Asia, having been cultivated for more than 5,000 years and has been known for its medicinal value. Sweet basil, maintained the year round in warm climates or in greenhouses, is easy to grow and maintain in containers.

Indian holy basil (*Ocimum sanctum*) is commonly known as *tulsi*. In India, this plant

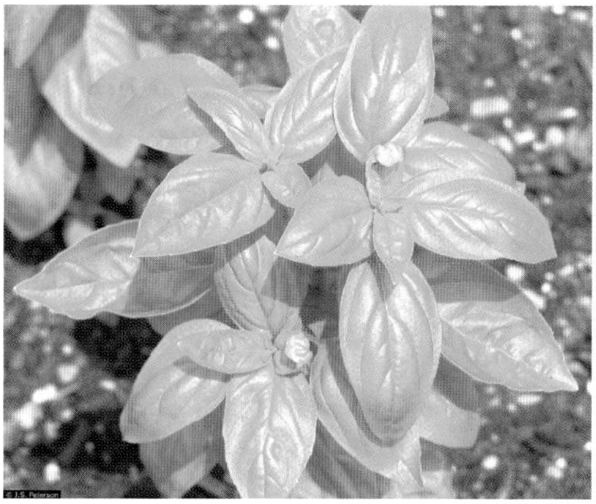

is an important Hindu religious symbol and is a primary herb in Ayurvedic treatment. The plant's extracts can be used to prevent and cure many ailments such as common cold, headaches, inflammation, stomach disorders, heart disease and malaria.

THYME (*Thymus vulgaris*) and LEMON THYME (*Thymus x citriodorus*)

Common or garden thyme and lemon thyme are two of the most commonly used species of thyme. Historically, man has used thyme since recorded time. It came to North America with the first colonists as a food preservative and medicine. Thyme has antiseptic and disinfectant properties. Thyme is used as a substitute for salt as well as blended with other herbs. It is used to flavour soups, stuffing, casseroles and baked or sautéed vegetables.

Thyme's aromatic oil contains two compounds, thymol and carvacrol, the source of its medicinal value. As a pharmaceutical, the oil is used in mouthwashes, toothpastes, soaps, liniments, throat lozenges, cough syrups and cold remedies. Because thyme is strongly antiseptic, it has traditionally been used as a remedy for respiratory infections. It has been suggested that drinking a cup of thyme tea three times a day eases sinus pain. To make thyme tea, steep 5 to 10 ml of dried thyme in 250 ml of boiling water for about ten minutes.

Thyme is an aromatic perennial shrub. Common thyme forms a dense mound, growing about 30 cm wide and tall. Flowers are lilac to pink and occur in June and July. Lemon thyme has a distinct lemon fragrance and is used for ornamental as well as culinary features. It forms a small 30 cm mound with small pale lilac flowers that are very similar to common garden thyme. It prefers well-drained soil.

Thyme can be grown in various types of containers. To increase the yield of each plant, clip it back after the first bloom. This produces an abundance of new stems that provide fresh cuttings for drying and a second bloom in late summer.

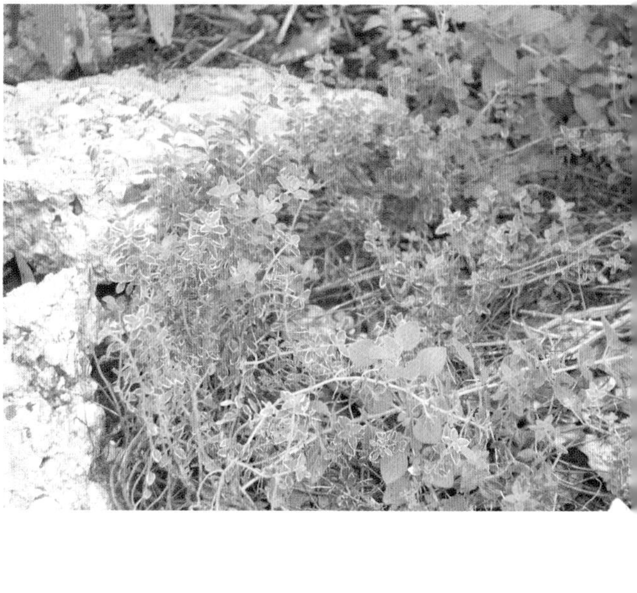

Ajwain (*Trachyspermum copticum*) is a plant native to India and is commonly used in Indian cuisine in pastries, snacks and breads. It contains the oil thymol and thus has a similar fragrance as thyme; it also has similar medicinal properties.

TEA TREE OIL (*Melaleuca alternifolia*)

The British explorer Captain James Cook first set foot in Australia in 1777. There he found the native people, the Aborigines, treating skin infections with crushed tea tree leaves. Today, tea tree oil is an ingredient in antiseptic creams and many other anti-microbial products.

The essential oil is released by crushing the leaves. It is a powerful antiseptic killing many micro-organisms that can cause infections, including yeast, fungus and bacteria that are penicillin resistant. Tea tree oil is also used to treat athlete's foot and stubborn, hard-to-treat fungal infected toenails. Use a cotton swap to apply 100 per cent tea tree oil to affected skin or toenails twice a day. For applying to sensitive skin of small children, the oil should be diluted in vegetable oil before applying to the skin. Although tea tree oil is safe for skin applications, it should never be taken internally because it is very toxic if swallowed.

Native to the moist areas on the northern coast of New South Wales and southern Queensland, Australia, tea tree is an evergreen that can grow to more than 10 metres. It has narrow, needle-like leaves and produces white flowers that bloom in summer.

TURMERIC (*Curcuma longa*)

This bright yellow spice is most commonly known as turmeric. It is known as *ukon* to the Japanese, *jiang huang* to the Chinese, *haldi* in India, and mistakenly as 'Indian saffron' in other areas of the world. Turmeric is a close botanical relative of ginger. The stalk of the plant is regularly used in both herbal and traditional medicine and provides a distinctive yellow-orange colour to any curry.

In addition to its role in cooking, the herb held a place of honour in India's traditional

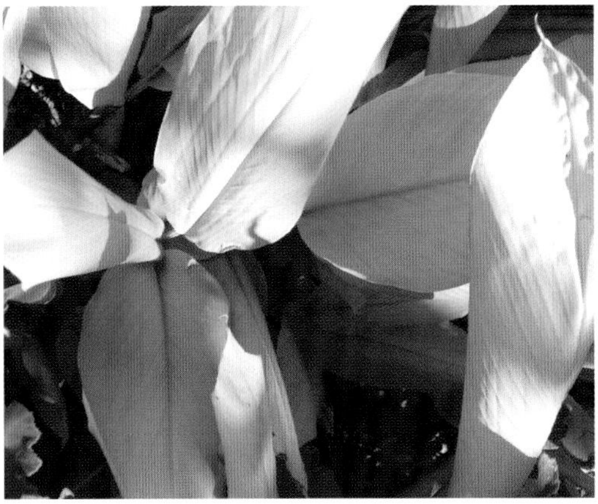

Ayurvedic medicine. Medically it was used as a digestive aid and as a treatment for fever, infection, dysentery, arthritis and jaundice or other liver ailments. Traditional Chinese physicians prescribed turmeric to treat liver and gallbladder problems, stop bleeding and relieve chest congestion. The ancient Greeks were well aware of turmeric. However, unlike its close botanical relative ginger, it never caught on in the West as a medicinal herb until recently.

Due to lack of interest by Western scientists and herbalists, the vast majority of research involving this herb has been conducted in India. Curcumin, the yellow pigment in turmeric, is the most medicinally active compound. Curcumin is an immune stimulant that exhibits anti-microbial and anti-inflammatory properties. It also soothes the stomach and provides liver and heart-protecting action. Turmeric stimulates the flow of bile. Bile helps digest fats. The German Commission E approves turmeric for indigestion.

Turmeric is not a garden herb in North America. It is chiefly cultivated in Southeast Asia as a perennial. It produces a tuberous rhizome (underground stem) that grows to roughly two feet (0.6 m) in length. It grows to a height of approximately one metre. The plant has large leaves, a central flower spike and funnel-shaped yellow flowers.

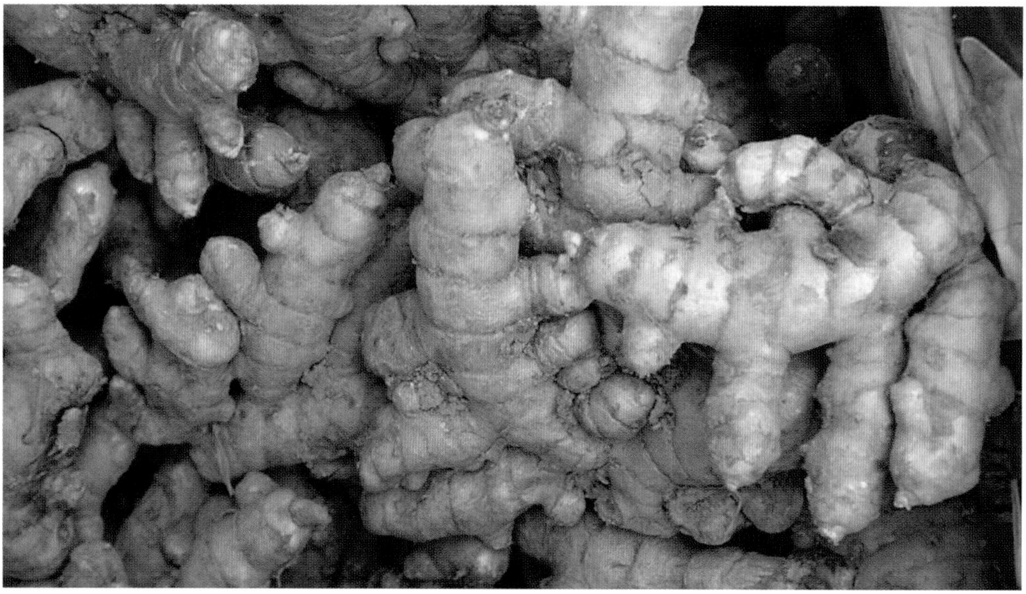

WINTER CHERRY or ASHWAGANDHA ROOT (*Withania somnifera*)

A native of India, Pakistan and Sri Lanka, *ashwagandha* is among the most prominent herbal preparations used in traditional Ayurvedic medicine. The plant contains molecules that are steroidal and it has active ingredients of Asian ginseng (*Panax ginseng*). Some know the plant as 'Indian ginseng'. Studies have shown its steroid content to be more potent than hydrocortisone, used to treat arthritis pain and inflammation in animals and humans. Thus it is often prescribed to inhibit inflammation. Studies by American psychiatrists found that the herb is also effective in the treatment of manic depression, alcohol paranoia and schizophrenia. It is often prescribed to increase the body's resistance to physical and emotional stress.

The plant is a low-lying perennial shrub having small greenish yellow flowers. The dried root is usually used to make a tea that is consumed up to three times a day. No significant side effects have been reported but it should not be taken during pregnancy.

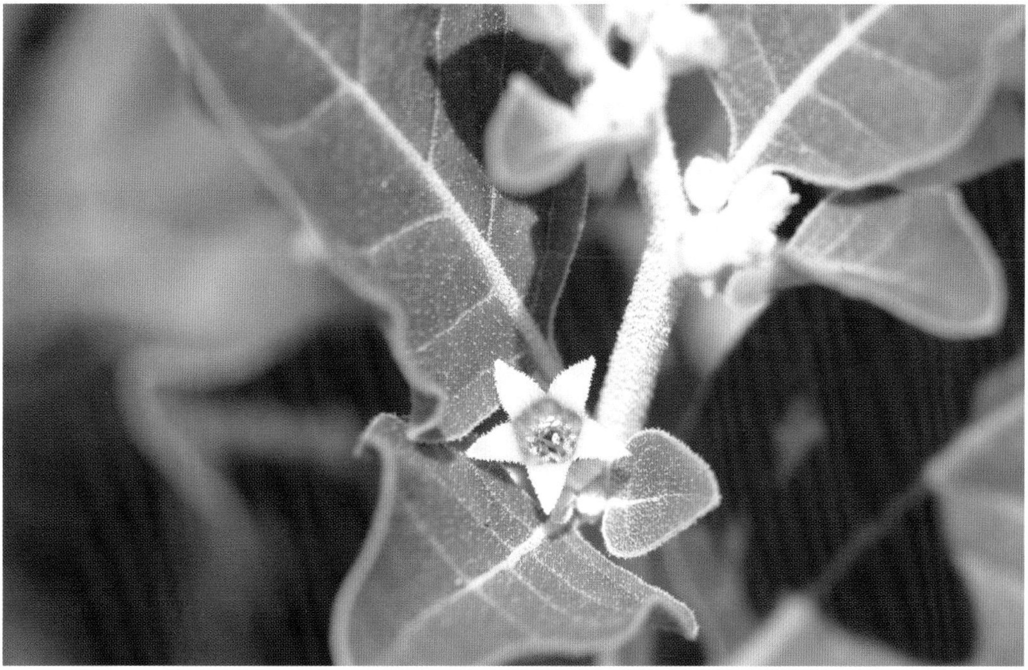

AROMATHERAPY

Aromatherapy means 'treatment using scents'. It is the use of essential oils to enhance human health and well-being. Essential oils are highly concentrated substances extracted from various parts of aromatic plants and trees. These aromatic plants and oils have been used since the beginning of the history of humankind. The Greeks, Romans, Egyptians and Chinese all used essential oils during their early history. Hippocrates, a Greek physician who is considered the 'Father of Western Medicine', used essential oils for aromatic baths and scented massages more than 2,000 years ago. He also used aromatic fumigation to rid Athens of the plague.

The modern era of aromatherapy began during the early 1900s when a French chemist named René-Maurice Gattefossé first used the name aromatherapy for the therapeutic use of essential oils. Aromatherapy is a holistic treatment of the body with pleasant-smelling botanical oils such as rose, lemon, lavender, eucalyptus, peppermint, chamomile, frankincense, etc. Aromatherapy is used for pain relief, for the care for the skin, to alleviate fatigue and to invigorate the entire body.

There are about 200 essential oils and most have antiseptic properties. Other properties of these oils are stimulation, relaxation and digestive improvements. To get maximum benefit from essential oils, they should be extracted from pure, raw plants, not those that have been synthesized from chemical sources. The essential oils are added to the bath or massaged into the skin, inhaled directly or diffused to scent an entire room. When inhaled, they work on the brain and nervous system. They act to stimulate the olfactory nerves and the part of the brain that controls emotion.

Aromatherapy became less popular in the Western world during the mid-1900s when the prescription drug industry began to develop synthetic counterparts to natural aromatic oils. However, today, due to the toxic side effects of many synthetic medications, aromatherapy is one of the fastest growing fields in alternative medicine. It is widely used in homes, clinics and hospitals for a variety of applications.

In Japan, some new buildings make use of aroma systems. In one commercial building, the scents of lavender and rosemary are pumped into the customer area to help calm customers who are waiting in line. In a bank, the scents of lemon and eucalyptus are released to help increase the alertness of its employees.

According to an article (8 December 2006) in the *Japanese Times*, 'doctors are turning to aromatherapy for help.' Dr Kazunaga Kawabata, who heads a clinic in Suita, Osaka Prefecture, began to look for alternative treatments for individuals with poor blood circulation as well as other medical problems about a decade ago. He found, through a series of experiments, that fragrant substances are absorbed through the skin and lungs into the blood vessels, causing various pharmacological reactions.

TOP 10 ESSENTIAL OILS *		
Common Name	**Botanical name**	**Benefits**
Eucalyptus	*Eucalyptus globules* or *Eucalyptus radiata*	Helpful in treating respiratory problems, such as coughs, cold and asthma. Also helps to boost the immune system, and relieve muscle tension.
Ylang Ylang	*Cananga odorata*	Helps one relax, and can reduce muscle tension. Good antidepressant.
Geranium	*Pelargonium graveolens*	Helps balance hormones in women; good for the skin. Can be both relaxing and uplifting and works as an antidepressant.
Peppermint	*Mentha piperita*	Useful in treating headaches, muscle aches, digestive disorders such as slow digestion, indigestion and flatulence.
Lavender	*Lavandula angustifolia*	Relaxing; also useful in treating wounds, burns, and used for skin care.
Lemon	*Citrus limon*	Very uplifting, yet relaxing. Helpful in treating wounds, infections, and house-cleaning and deodorizing.
Clary Sage	*Salvia sclarea*	Natural painkiller, helpful in treating muscular aches and pains. Very relaxing, and can help with insomnia. Also very helpful in balancing hormones.
Tea Tree Oil	*Melaleuca alternifolia*	A natural antifungal oil, good for treating all sorts of infections including vaginal yeast infections, jock itch, athelete's foot and ringworm. Also helps boost the immune system.
Roman Chamomile	*Anthemis nobilis*	Very relaxing, and can help with sleeplessness and anxiety. Also good for muscle aches and tension. Useful in treating wounds and infection.
Rosemary	*Rosmarinus officinalis*	Very stimulating and uplifting, good to help mental stimulation as well as to stimulate the immune system. Very good for muscle aches and tension. Stimulating to the digstive system.

* *Source: National Association for Holistic Aromatherapy (http://www.naha.org)*

Plants: Their Role in Water and Waste Recycling

Water is an essential element in the life processes of all plants, animals and humans. Fortunately, water is also earth's most abundant resource, covering approximately three-fourths of the earth's surface. About 97 per cent of this water is found in the oceans and is too salty for drinking or other uses. The remaining 3 per cent is fresh water. About three-fourths of that amount is frozen in icecaps and other glaciers. Groundwater makes up most of the remaining amount and is available in most parts of the world. However, some groundwater is so deep underground as to make it cost-prohibitive to extract. Less than 0.1 per cent of all available fresh water remains for lakes, creeks, streams, rivers and rainfall. This is the water that must be used again and again.

Globally, the total volume of water is essentially constant and is one of earth's most renewable resources. A large portion of fresh water is continually collected as water vapour and distributed by nature's hydrologic cycle. Eventually, all water on earth passes through the atmosphere as water vapour. It is then returned to earth in the form of precipitation.

One large tree can add more than 200 gallons (0.75 cubic m) of water to the ambient atmosphere each day. Therefore, forests and green spaces in all regions of the world play a vital role in nature's water cycle. Evaporation and plant transpiration also remove salts and other impurities added by nature and human activity, making it possible to reuse the same water indefinitely. This natural water cycle produces sufficient quantities of fresh water, provided it is neither contaminated nor used more rapidly than it can replenish itself.

As essential as water is to life, it is not evenly distributed over the earth. Through actions of the hydrologic cycle, fresh water supplies separate the earth into tropical and temperate zones and arid and semi-arid zones. The water supply of a region is determined by its precipitation. If rainfall were evenly distributed, all land would receive an estimated 34 inches (0.86 m) of rain annually. In fact, one inch (2.5 cm) of rain provides 27,000 gallons (102 cubic m) of water per acre (0.4 hectare). However, north-eastern India averages more than 400 inches (10 m) per year while the northern region of Chile may not receive rain for several years.

Civilizations have necessarily populated areas that have an ample supply of fresh water. However, the world's burgeoning population (over 6 billion) has placed a tremendous stress on the water supply of some regions. According to WHO, more than one billion people – one sixth of the world's population – lack access to safe water supply.

Plants help to determine the type of climate that exists in a particular region of the world. Removal of vast expanses of trees and other vegetation can contribute to climate change and in some cases cause the formation of deserts. Currently, there is world tension over the limited supply of energy – oil and natural gas. But the World Bank has sounded an alarm regarding the lack of water in the Middle East and parts of Africa as the water shortage worsens each day. Water shortages are also beginning to appear in heavily populated countries, such as India and China.

A major threat to our supply of fresh, clean water is pollution. Our fresh water supply comes from two sources: 1) surface waters (lakes, rivers and streams), and 2) underground aquifers.

Lake Baikal in southern Siberia in Russia is the world's oldest and deepest fresh water lake. Although it is smaller in surface area than the US/Canadian Great Lakes, it holds more water than all five Great Lakes combined. The combined volume of water in the Great Lakes and Lake Baikal holds an estimated 40 per cent of all fresh surface water on earth.

Most metropolitan areas obtain their drinking water from surface waters. Yet, 40 per cent of US waters do not meet basic water quality standards. Surface water pollution is generally categorized as resulting from point sources and non-point sources. Point sources of pollution are discharges from a specific source such as an industrial or chemical complex or a wastewater treatment system. Non-point sources, as the name implies, have no specific discharge point, but would include urban storm water runoff, runoff from agricultural or mining operations, construction sites, landfill leachates and toxic chemical spills. The EPA estimates that as much as 65 per cent of surface water pollutants come from non-point sources.

Underground aquifers are the source of about half of all of our drinking water. The source for much of the water used to recharge the aquifers is from agricultural runoff. These waters often contain excessive amounts of insecticides, herbicides and fertilizers.

One of the more promising solutions to our water pollution problems is as old as the earth itself and was used by our ancestors. Phytoremediation is a promising natural biotechnology that is cost effective and environmentally friendly. Phytoremediation is simply a process that uses human and animal waste as a food source for plants and their root-associated microbes with the ultimate goal of purifying the wastewater as it slowly flows through plant root zones.

PLANTS AND RECYCLING WASTE

In nature's basic form, human and animal waste sustains plants by supplying them with the essential nutrients for growth. In other words, these waste products are nature's perfect organic fertilizer. In most Asian countries, the method of using waste for plant growth has been practised for thousands of years. Organic fertilizers produce highly productive soil, making it sustainable for an indefinite period of time. Not only can organic fertilizer be used to grow food crops but its use can support plant growth for other applications while treating human and animal waste.

Although Asian countries have used human waste, also referred to as night soil, on gardens and fields for centuries, this practice was never accepted in the Western world since night soil produces offensive odours and provides a route of transmission for various pathogenic micro-organisms, especially parasites, when applied openly to soil surfaces. On the other hand, when the same soil is continuously farmed with synthetic fertilizers, trace minerals necessary for plant growth are depleted. Organic fertilizers contain sufficient quantities of nitrogen, phosphorus, potassium and trace elements to continuously renew the soil. Now that earth's population continues to increase and available farmland decreases, the Western world is faced with a dilemma.

When the American zoologist, Dr Edward Morse arrived in Tokyo in 1877, he was amazed to learn that its mortality rate was lower than that of Boston. Investigating the reasons, he noticed that there were few cases of dysentery, cholera or malaria. In short, Japan did not generally have diseases that were spread by poor sanitation. During the Edo Period (early seventeenth century to late nineteenth century), cholera outbreaks had occurred only when foreign ships put into port. In his book, *Japan Day by Day* (1917), Morse attributed the lack of these types of diseases to the fact that all human waste was carried away from the city by farmers and used as fertilizer to grow food crops. He observed that in America, by contrast, untreated sewage flowed into bays and inlets, contaminating water and killing marine life. Conditions were the same or worse in Europe.

Beginning in Japan about 1649, the dumping from toilets of raw human excreta (night soil) directly into rivers and moats was forbidden. Around 1856 farmers began carting off night soil to use as fertilizer. Thanks to this cycle, sewage systems were not needed, even in the cities. As a result, the waterways were not contaminated by waste and drinking water did not transmit diseases.

Dr F.H. King authored a book in 1910 entitled *Farmers of Forty Centuries*. Dr King, a former chief of the Division of Soil Management of the US Department of Agriculture, travelled through Japan, Korea and China in the early 1900s as an agricultural visitor. He sought to understand how the Asian people could farm the same fields for thousands of years without destroying the soil's fertility. He discovered that the practice of applying human and animal waste to the soils kept it fertile. Today, we call this practice 'sustainable agriculture'.

In 1952, the Chinese recycled about 70 per cent of their night soil. The practice increased to almost 90 per cent by 1956 and constituted about one-third of all fertilizers in China. However, today they have mostly abandoned the practice. Between the mid-1960s and mid-1980s, China increased its use of synthetic fertilizers more than 600 per cent. By 1992, an estimated 45 billion tonnes of mostly untreated wastewater flowed annually into China's rivers and lakes. Water pollution is now one of China's biggest environmental problems. India has similar pollution problems. According to UNICEF, India has the greatest proportion of people in the world, other than Nepal, without access to improved sanitation.

There are promising methods on the horizon that could turn some of these environmental liabilities into assets in China and India. Technology is available that could reduce the volume of wastewater that currently enters their rivers and streams. One possible method is that wastewater is pumped to large lagoons on the outskirts of cities. By placing floating covers over the lagoons, methane gas is produced as the waste solids are anaerobically (without oxygen) digested by micro-organisms. The methane gas is collected and stored. The nutrient-enriched wastewater is pumped via pipelines to distribution points in the rural farmland. Farmers then haul the liquid fertilizer to their farms and apply it to the soil. In this way, the soil would become much more fertile and the local rivers and streams would receive much less waste. The concept is not complicated, would be cost-effective and more importantly go a long way toward solving water pollution problems in China, India and other countries. Generally, this method or other similar approaches need to be applied on a small scale to prove its economic viability before large-scale operations are employed.

In the past the use of waste as a fertilizer has been unsanitary and, in some cases, has led to the spread of diseases. Bodily wastes have all the elements necessary to sustain some viruses and bacteria and may contain pathogenic microbes. For this reason, precautions are necessary whenever waste is used as a fertilizer. New hydroponic growing methods use human waste in a more sanitary manner and eliminate health risks by avoiding human contact with untreated waste. A significant problem in using these techniques is overcoming the negative connotations related to the use of human waste. Western nations have immense psychological compunction regarding the use of untreated human and animal waste as fertilizer. It is always best to work in harmony with nature to solve our environmental pollution problems.

NASA Studies the Role of Plants in Waste Recycling

NASA began to study methods of waste recycling for use in long-term space habitation in the early 1970s. Disposing of human waste products is obviously a much more difficult undertaking in space than here on earth. NASA's Stennis Space Center (SSC) in Mississippi began by studying human urine as a hydroponic nutrient solution for growing food plants. Hydroponic growing methods generally do not use soil and a nutrient solution flows past the plants' root systems at periodic intervals.

Urine from a healthy person is sterile, that is, free of micro-organisms. It is made up of approximately 95 per cent water, 2.5 per cent urea (a nitrogen compound) and 2.5 per cent a mixture of minerals and organic substances such as hormones, amino acids, enzymes, etc. When diluted with water, urine makes an excellent fertilizer. To show the value of urine as a fertilizer, NASA scientists grew vegetables such as cherry tomatoes and green beans using a hydroponic solution consisting of 0.5 per cent urine and 99.5 per cent tap water.

In this study, a small electrical pump set on a timer pumped the urine/tap water solution from a holding tank past the root systems of numerous cherry tomato plants. The timer was set to pump for fifteen minutes every hour on a twenty-four-hour cycle. The urine/tap water solution was depleted through plant uptake and evapotranspiration. As a result, scientists added approximately 10 litres of the solution every seventh day. Liquid from the holding tank recycled through the system and was never discharged. The water that was transpired by the plants was clean, and thus, no pollutants entered the environment.

After a four-month period, the cherry tomato plants produced an average of 210 tomatoes per vine and had grown to a height of approximately 11 feet (3.4 m). The plants grew an average of one inch (2.5 cm) per day (see Fig. 6.1).

In a second study, scientists grew cherry tomatoes and green beans in a similar hydroponic system with the exception that domestic wastewater provided the nutrient source in this case. Standard plant nursery containers were filled with inert materials (small gravel and oyster shells) to hold the plants in place. A reservoir containing 10.58 gallons (40 litres) of domestic wastewater provided nutrients to the plants. Results similar to the urine solution study are evidenced in Fig. 6.2. Not only did the plants yield fruit, but analyses showed that

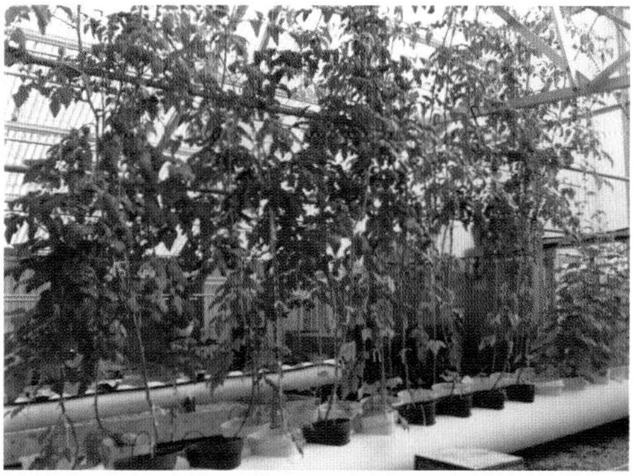

FIG. 6.1

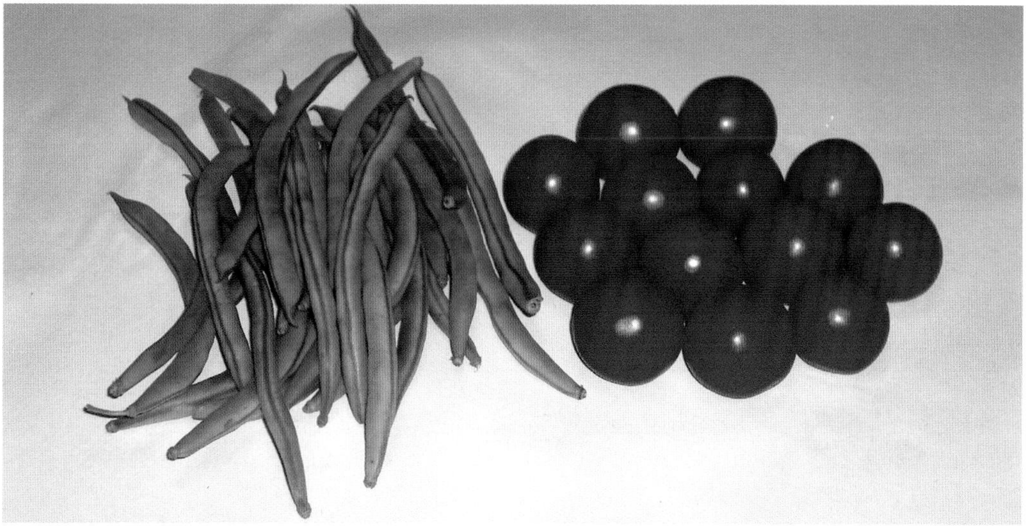

FIG. 6.2

significant wastewater treatment also took place (see Table 6.1).

Standard wastewater treatment analyses were made every seven days and included: BOD_5 (amount of oxygen removed from water during a five-day period); TSS (total suspended solids); NH_3 (ammonia nitrogen) and TP (total phosphorus).

TABLE 6.1

Test Parameter	Average Influent (mg/l)	Average Effluent (mg/l)
BOD_5	203	2.3
TSS	57	2.3
NH_3	18	<0.42
TP	3.9	0.96

These studies proved two important points: 1) Food crops will yield fruit when domestic wastewater is the only food source, and 2) advanced wastewater treatment can take place in as few as seven days.

The goals of NASA's plant research project at SSC were threefold: 1) To develop an immediate cost-effective method to treat chemical and domestic wastewater at SSC; 2) To develop bio-technology for use in future manned space habitats; and 3) To demonstrate 'spin-off' technology for solving the earth's environmental pollution problems.

In 1971, SSC researchers began to evaluate aquatic and semi-aquatic plants and their root microbes for their ability to cleanse wastewater. Pilot studies first used floating aquatic plants, such as water hyacinths (*Eichhornia crassipes*) and duckweed (*Lemna* sp.), in troughs filled with domestic wastewater. The successful results of these tests led to similar studies using various rooted plants, including bulrush (*Scirpus* sp.), cattails (*Typha latifolia*), reeds (*Phragmites communis*), canna lilies (*Canna flaccida*) and elephant ears or taro (*Colocasia esculenta*) among other plant species.

During a ten-year period, repetitive studies were conducted using small rock/plant filters and various plants to treat domestic wastewater. Each trough was filled to a depth of 7 inches (17.8 cm) with railroad ballast and a 2 inch (5.1 cm) top layer of small pea gravel. A continuous depth of approximately 7 inches (17.8 cm) of domestic wastewater was maintained in each trough (see Fig. 6.3).

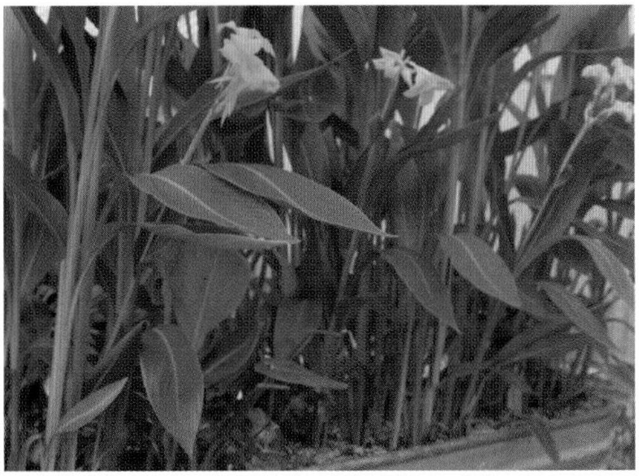

FIG. 6.3

The successful wastewater treatment results can be seen in the following chart:

TABLE 6.2
WASTEWATER TREATMENT BY REEDS
(*Phragmites communis*)

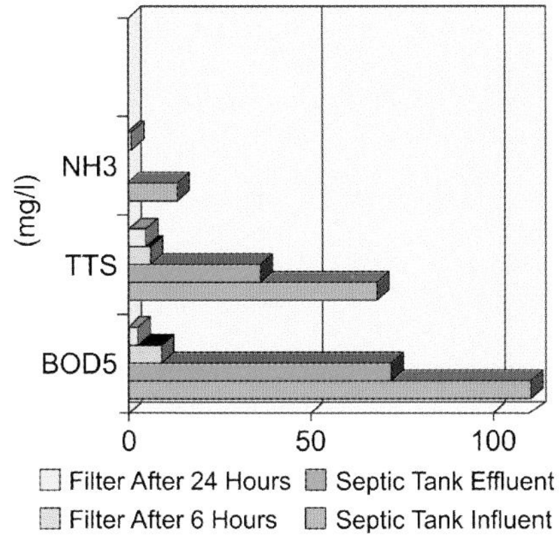

Beginning in 1974, all wastewater by the approximately 5,500 employees at SSC is treated in various phytoremediation systems using aquatic and semi-aquatic plants. These systems range from plant filters treating septic tank effluents at the reception centres to much larger systems treating waste from lagoons. As a result of NASA's research and early implementation of phytoremediation technologies, many small towns and cities in Mississippi and other Southern states employ these systems to treat their domestic wastewater.

Over the years, many subsequent applications and further development of the technology have occurred. For example, Douglas White, an innovative architect who lives in the dry, mountainous area on the island of St Thomas (US Virgin Islands), has used his creative talents to work in harmony with nature. In this part of the island, fresh water is a scarce commodity. He designed a hydroponic system for his home in which effluent from a septic tank is piped underneath the roots of a landscaped bed of shrubs and flowers. The dark, nutrient enriched, odorous liquid from the septic tank is deodorized and purified as it slowly filters through the system while supplying the plants with their primary source of food and water (see Fig. 6.4).

When properly designed and with sufficient contact time in the landscaped beds, plants and their root microbes can remove pollutants from the waste stream. This process is accepted throughout the world due to its sanitary attributes as the

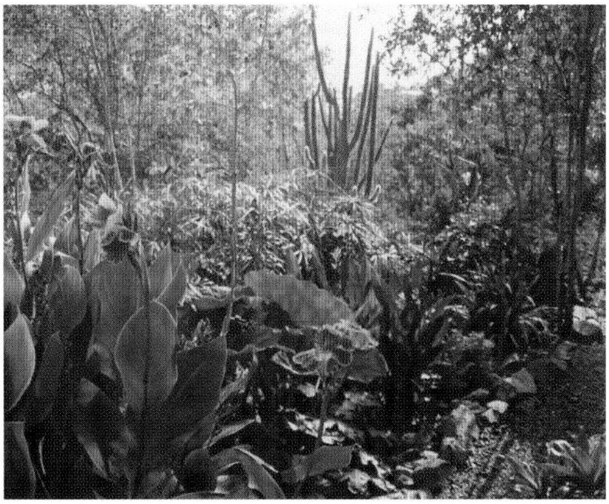

FIG. 6.4

odorous human waste remains underground and is never seen or smelled. It is a safe, environmentally friendly way to not only treat wastewater but to conserve water. To the casual observer, the visible effect is that of a lush garden and none would suspect that wastewater treatment is effectively taking place below or that it is the primary source of water and nutrients for the plants.

Environmentally conscious industries have sought out the technology as a way to provide final polishing of their chemical and industrial wastewater before releasing it into the environment. Two shining examples are cited here. Degussa Corporation operates a large chemical manufacturing complex in Theodore, Alabama. In 1988, they had constructed a phytoremediation system to act as a final polishing filter of their chemical wastewater before releasing it into the environmentally sensitive waters of Mobile Bay. The system has consistently provided effective treatment for almost twenty years (see Fig. 6.5.).

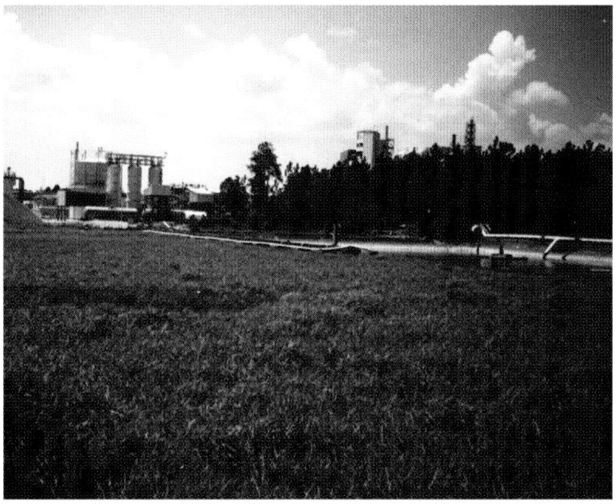

FIG. 6.5

Albemarle Corporation's two chemical manufacturing plants located in Magnolia, Arkansas also use marsh filters to treat process water and storm water runoff. The systems have proven so successful that Albemarle employees regularly conduct sight-seeing and educational tours in what has become a wildlife sanctuary (see Fig. 6.6).

Many different versions of phytoremediation or constructed wetland systems for treating wastewater have been developed and implemented throughout the world in recent years. In 2001, a book entitled *Growing Clean Water – Nature's Solution to Water Pollution* was published by Wolverton Environmental Services, Inc. This book details more than twenty-five years of research by Dr B.C. Wolverton on the use of plant-based filters for treating both industrial and domestic wastewater. Operational data on many wastewater treatment systems using NASA-derived biotechnology is displayed in this book.

These successful systems are important to prove the vital role that plants play in cleaning and recycling our limited supply of fresh water. In nature, plants act to filter, trap and assimilate impurities with which they

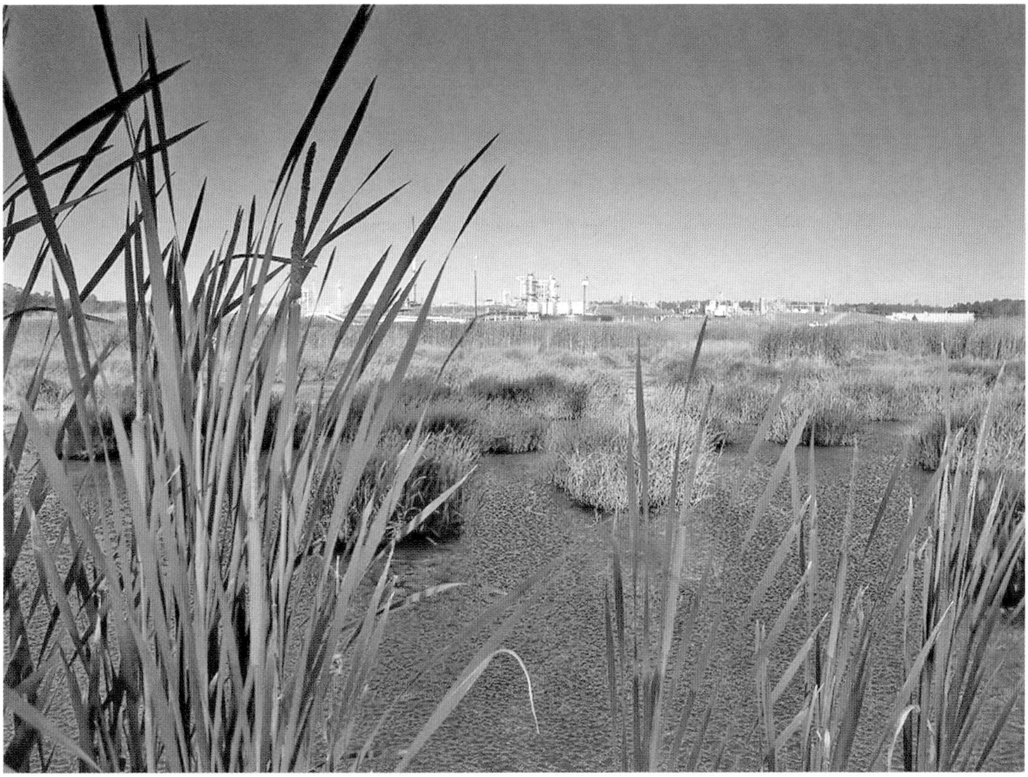

FIG. 6.6

come in contact. It only makes sense that we use our engineering expertise to aid plants in their efforts to clean the pollutants human activity adds to our environment.

Phytofilters for Treating Industrial Air Pollution

A very promising concept makes use of phytofilters in the treatment of industrial air pollution from a single source, that is, smokestacks, incinerators, etc. The process converts the air pollutant into water pollutants and then treats the water with a phytofilter. Electrical power generation plants that burn high-sulphur coal (dirty coal), waste incinerators and animal factory farms are also possible applications for this process. Animal factory farms are large operations housing poultry, swine, cattle, etc., in confined facilities, thus generating noxious odours and voluminous animal waste products. An artist's concept depicting a swine/poultry facility where both the air and wastewater are treated in a phytofilter system is shown in Fig. 6.7.

Countries such as the US, China, Russia, India and Australia have large reserves of coal, a relatively inexpensive energy source. However, most of the coal contains high concentrations of sulphur. Burning high-sulphur coal produces exhaust gases that are usually above acceptable levels of pollution. Because of the harm these exhaust gases cause to our environment, regulatory agencies and the general public continue to pressure companies against the use of high-sulphur coal. If a method were available to strip the pollutants from the exhaust gases before they were released into the air, a bountiful energy supply would be more readily accessible for power generation.

ODOUR CONTROL AND WASTEWATER TREATMENT SYSTEM FOR SWINE/POULTRY OPERATIONS

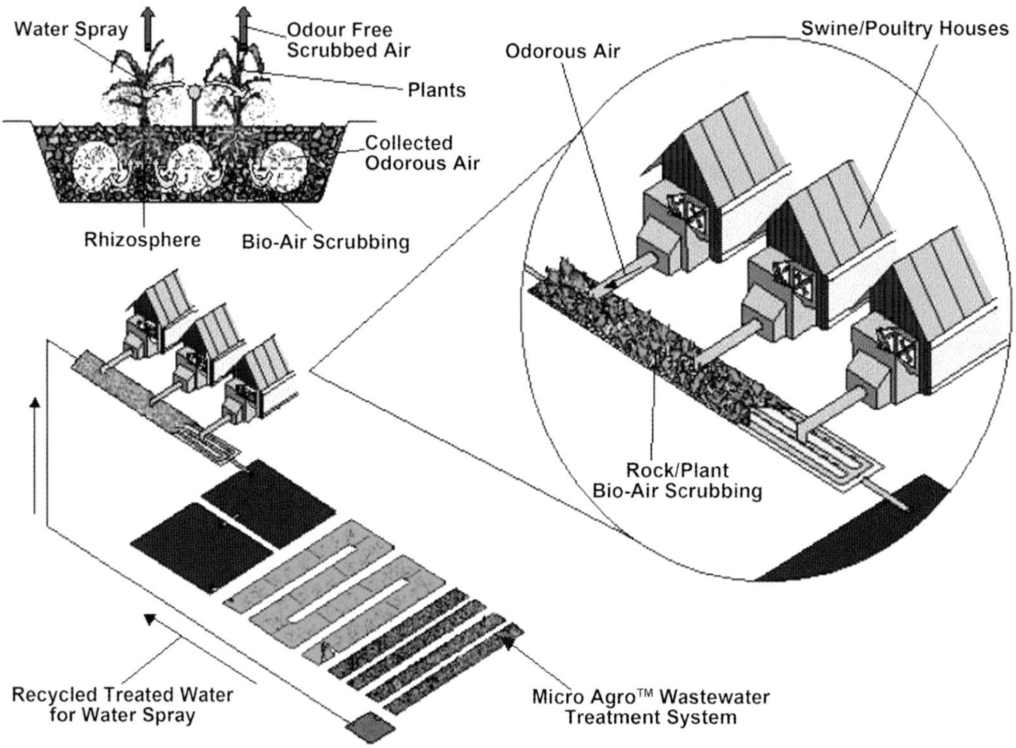

FIG. 6.7

Small-scale studies on the treatment of air pollution emanating from incinerators have been conducted by WES. These studies have shown the potential of using wet scrubber technology to convert air pollution into water pollution. The polluted water then slowly flows through a phytofilter (constructed wetlands) where plants break down the pollutants into useable sources of food and thus, clean the water. The water is then recycled for use in the wet scrubber process. Although the pilot-scale system was successful, it is yet to be proven whether a scale-up in the technology is feasible in a large-scale operation.

The future is filled with exciting new applications that plants and their root-associated microbes can play to enhance our lives and sustain our environment. It is sometimes just a matter of 'thinking outside the box' or a willingness to try things that have not been done before. We humans are creative by nature and bold in thought. Nature, even in its rawest form, is a powerful force. When nature is harnessed with man's technological ingenuity, the possibilities are endless. Therefore, optimism abounds that we will continue to look for new ways in which we can work in harmony with nature to provide a bright future for generations to come.

References

CHAPTER 1: IS THE AIR INDOORS MAKING YOU SICK?

Beasley, R., et al., 'The global burden of asthma report,' Medical Research Institute of New Zealand and the University of Southampton (UK) in association with the Global Initiative for Asthma, May 2004.

Burkhard, C., 'Chemical emissions from office equipment,' *IVF Research Publication* 99826, 1999.

CDC Morbidity and Mortality Weekly Report (MMWR), 24 April 1998, 47(53:1), 1-28, 'Surveillance for asthma – US 1960-1995.'

'Common Indoor Air Pollutants – Biological Contaminants,' Available from http://www.prohousedr.com/mold.htm (17 February 2003); INTERNET.

Fisk, W.J., 'Health and productivity gains from better indoor environments and their relationship with building energy efficiency,' *Annual Review of Energy and the Environment*, 2000, 25(1):1-30.

Fisk, W.J., 'Review of health and productivity gains from better IEQ,' Proceedings of *Healthy Buildings* 2000 (Helsinki), Vol. 4, pp. 23-24.

Fisk, W.J. and A.H. Rosenfeld, 'Estimates of improved productivity and health from better indoor environments,' *Indoor Air*, 1997, 7:158-172.

Friebele, E., 'The Attack of Asthma,' *Environmental Health Perspectives*, Jan. 1996, Vol. 104(1): 22-25.

'Global Burden of Asthma' (May 2004), Global Initiative for Asthma (GINA). Available from http://www.ginasthma.org.

'IAQ Fact Sheet – Biological Contaminants,' National Safety Council – Environmental Health Center, March 2000. Available from http://www.nsc.org/ehc/indoor/bio_cont.htm (17 February 2003); INTERNET.

'Indoor Air Quality: Biological Contaminants,' Available from http://www.nutramed.com/environment/handbook-bio.htm (17 February 2003); INTERNET.

Magill, M.K. and A. Suruda, 'Multiple chemical sensitivity syndrome,' *American Family Physician*, 1 September 1998.

Pezzoli, G., et al., 'Hydrocarbon exposure and Parkinson's disease,' *Neurology*, 2000, 55:667-673.

Rumchev, K., et al. 'Association of domestic exposure to volatile organic compounds with asthma in young children,' *Thorax*, 2004, 59:746-751.

Samet, J.M. and John D. Spengler (eds.), *Indoor Air Pollution a Health Perspective*, John Hopkins University Press, Baltimore, 1991.

'Surveillance for Asthma – U.S. 1960-1995,' CDC Morbidity and Mortality Weekly Report (MMWR), 24 April 1998, 47(SS-1); 1-28.

'Toxic trailer issue passed around,' *The Sun Herald*, Biloxi, Mississippi, 31 May 2007.

US Environmental Protection Agency. *Indoor Air Facts No. 4 (revised): Sick Building Syndrome* (SBS) (April 1991).

US Environmental Protection Agency, Office of Air and Radiation. Report to Congress on *Indoor Air Quality, Volume II: Assessment and Control of Indoor Air Pollution*, pp. 1, 4-14. EPA-400-1-89-001C, 1989.

US Environmental Protection Agency Report to Congress. *Indoor Air Quality in Public Buildings*: Vols. I and II (1988) EPA/00/6-88/009ab.

US Environmental Protection Agency Report to Congress. *Indoor Air Quality: Executive Summary and Recommendations* (1989) EPA/400/1-89/001A.

'U.S. rules allow the sale of products others ban,' *Los Angeles Times*, 8 October 2006.

Wensing, M., 'Determination of organic chemical emissions from electronic devices,' G. Raw, C. Aizlewood, and O. Warren (eds.), *Proceedings of the 8th International Conference on Indoor Air and Climate*, Edinburg, UK, 1999, Vol. 5, pp. 87-92.

Wolverton, B.C. *How To Grow Fresh Air, Penguin*, New York, 1997; first published in the United Kingdom as *Eco-Friendly Houseplants*, Weidenfeld & Nicolson Ltd., London, 1996.

CHAPTER 2: PLANTS: NATURE'S AIR PURIFIERS

Axcell, B.C. and P.J. Geary, 'Purification and some properties of a soluble benzene-oxidizing system from a strain of *Pseudomonas,' Biochem. J.*, 1975, 146: 173-183.

Davies, J.K. and W.C. Evans, 'Oxidation metabolism of naphthalene by soil *Pseudomonads,' Biochem. J.*, 1964, 91: 251-264.

Di Justo, Patrick, 'The 54-Story Air Filter,' *Popular Science*, Vol. 266, #3 (March 2005), pp. 28-29.

Evans, W.C., H.N. Fernley and E. Griffith, 'Oxidation metabolism of phenanthrene and anthracene by soil *Pseudomonads,' Biochem. J.*, 1965, 95: 809-813.

Giese, M., U. Bauer-Doranth, C. Langebartels and H. Sandermann, Jr., 'Detoxification of formaldehyde by the spider plant (*Chlorophytum comosum L.*) cell suspension cultures,' *Plant Physiology*, 1994, 104: 1301-1309.

Karns, J.S., S. Duttagupta and A.M. Chakrabarty, 'Regulation of 2,4,5-trichlorophenoxyacetic acid and chlorophenol metabolism in *Pseudomonas cepacia* AC1100,' *Appl. Environ. Microbiol.*, 1983, 46: 1182-1186.

La Pat-Polasko, L.T., P.L. McCarthy and A.J.B. Zehnder, 'Secondary substrate utilization of methylene chloride by an isolated strain of *Pseudomonas* sp.,' *Applied Environ. Microbiol.*, 1984, 47(4): 825-830.

Lohr, V.I. and C.H. Person-Mims, 'Particulate matter accumulation on horizontal surfaces in interiors: Influence of foliage plants,' *Atmospheric Environment*, 1996, 30(14): 2565-2568.

Tabak, H.H., et al., 'Biodegradability studies with organic priority pollutant compounds,' *J. Water Poll. Control Fed.*, 1981, 53(10): 1503-1518.

US Environmental Protection Agency Report to Congress, *Indoor Air Quality in Public Buildings*: Vols. I and II (1988) EPA/00/6-88-009ab.

Wolverton, B.C. and D.D. Harrison, 'Aquatic plants for removal of mevinphos from the aquatic environment,' *J. MS Acad. of Sci.*, 1973, 19: 84-88.

Wolverton, B.C., R.C. McDonald and E.A. Watkins, Jr., 'Foliage plants for removing indoor air pollutants from energy-efficient homes,' *Econ. Bot.*, 1984, 38(2): 224-228.

Wolverton, B.C., R.C. McDonald and H.H. Mesick, 'Foliage plants for the indoor removal of the primary combustion gases carbon monoxide and nitrogen oxides,' *J. MS Acad. of Sci.*, 1985, 30: 1-8.

Wolverton, B.C., R.C. McCaleb and W.L. Douglas, 'Bioregenerative space and terrestrial habitats,' Ninth Biennial Princeton Conf. on Space Mfg., Space Studies Institute, Princeton, NJ, 11 May 1989.

Wolverton, B.C., A. Johnson and K. Bounds, 'Interior landscape plants for indoor air pollution abatement,' NASA/ALCA Final Report, *Plants for Clean Air Council*, Mitchellville, MD, 1989.

Wolverton, B.C., 'Plants and their microbial assistants:

Nature's answer to earth's environmental pollution problems,' Biological Life Support Technologies: Commercial Opportunities, M. Nelson and G. Soffen (eds.), proceedings from a workshop sponsored by NASA, 1989.

Wolverton, B.C. and J. Wolverton, 'Bioregenerative life support systems for energy-efficient buildings,' Proceedings of Intl. Conf. of Life Support and Biospherics, Huntsville, AL, 1992.

Wolverton, B.C. and J. Wolverton, 'Removal of formaldehyde from sealed chambers by azalea, poinsettia and dieffenbachia,' Research Report No. WES/100/01-91/005, *Plants for Clean Air Council,* Mitchellville, MD, 1991.

Wolverton, J. and B.C. Wolverton, 'Improving indoor air quality using orchids and bromeliads,' Research Report No. WES/100/12-91/006, *Plants for Clean Air Council*, Mitchellville, MD, 1991.

Wolverton, B.C. and J.D. Wolverton, 'Interior plants and their role in indoor air quality: an overview,' Research Report No. WES/100/06-92/008, *Plants for Clean Air Council*, Mitchellville, MD, 1992.

Wolverton, B.C., 'Nature's answer to indoor air pollution,' Improving the Environment, proceedings of the Twelfth Annual Conf. and Expo. on Facility Mgmt., San Diego, CA, 10-13 Nov. 1991, pp. 270-281.

Wolverton, B.C. and J.D. Wolverton, 'Plants and soil micro-organisms – removal of formaldehyde, xylene and ammonia from the indoor environment,' *J. of the MS Acad. of Sci.*, 1993, 38(2): 11-15.

Wolverton, B.C., 'Can plants improve air quality in office environments?' Understanding the Workplace of Tomorrow, proceedings of the Fourteenth Annual Conf. and Expo. on Facility Mgmt., Denver, CO, 10-13 Oct. 1993, pp. 280-288.

Wolverton, B.C. *Eco-Friendly Houseplants*. Weidenfeld & Nicolson, London, 1996; Released in the US as *How To Grow Fresh Air*. Penguin, New York, 1997.

Wolverton, B.C. and J.D. Wolverton, 'Interior plants: their influence on airborne microbes inside energy-efficient buildings,' *J. of the MS Acad. of Sci.*, 1996, 41(2): 99-105.

Wood, R.A., et al., 'Study of absorption of VOCs by commonly used indoor plants,' proceedings of Indoor Air '99, 1999, 2: 690-694.

Wood, R.A., et al., 'Potted plant-growth media: interactions and capacities in removal of volatiles from indoor air,' *J of Environ. Hort. And Biotechnology,* 2002, 77(1): 120-129.

Wood, R.A., M.D. Burchett, et al., 'The potted-plant microcosm substantially reduces indoor air VOC pollution; I. Office Field-Study,' *J of Water, Air and Soil Pollution*, 2006, 175(1-4): 163-180.

CHAPTER 3: INTERIOR PLANTS FOR HUMAN HEALTH AND WELL-BEING

Arnold, J.W. and B.W. Mitchell, 'Use of negative air ionization for reducing microbial contamination on stainless steel surfaces,' *J. of Applied Poultry Research*, 2002, Vol. 11:179-186.

Fjeld, T., et al., 'Effect of indoor foliage plants on health and discomfort symptoms among office workers,' *Indoor + Build Environment*, 1998, 7: 204-206.

Fjeld, T., 'The effect of plants and artificial day-light on the well-being and health of office workers, school children and healthcare personnel,' Seminar Report: Reducing Health Complaints at Work, Plants for People, International Horticulture Exhibit, Floriade 2002 (Netherlands).

Gerlach-Spriggs, N., R.E. Kaufman and S.B. Warner, *Restorative Gardens: The Healing Landscape*, Yale University Press, 1998.

Kimura, S., M. Ashiba and I. Matsushima, 'Influences of the Air Lacking in Light Ions and the Effect of Its Artificial Ionization upon Human Beings in Occupied Rooms,' *Japanese Journal of Medical Science*, 1939, 7:1-12.

Kruger, A.P. and D.S. Sobel, 'Air ions and health,' *Ways*

of Health: Holistic Approach to Ancient and Contemporary Medicine, David S. Sobel (ed.), Harcourt Brace Jovanovich, New York, 1979, pp. 413-433.

Kruger, A.P. and S. Sheelth, 'Ions in the air,' *Human Nature*, 1 July 1978, pp. 46-52.

Kruger, A.P. and E.J. Reed, 'Biological impact of small ions,' *Science*, 1976, 193: 1209-1213.

Lohr, V.I., et al., 'Interior plants may improve worker productivity and reduce stress in a windowless environment,' J. Environ. Hort., 1996, 14: 97-100.

Lohr, V.I. and C.H. Person-Mims, 'Physical discomfort may be reduced in the presence of interior plants,' *Horticultural Technology*, 2000, 10(1): 53-58.

Lorh, V.I., 'The contribution of interior plants to relative humidity in an office,' D. Relf (ed.), *The Role of Horticulture in Human Well-Being and Social Development: A National Symposium*, Timber Press, 1992, 117-119.

Nakamura, R. and E. Fujii, 'Studies of the characteristics of the electroencephalogram when observing potted plants: *Pelargonium hortorum* "Sprinter Red" and *Begonia evansiana*,' *Technical Bulletin of the Faculty of Horticulture of Chiba University*, 1990, 43: 177-183.

Rolf, Diane (ed.), *The Role of Horticulture in Human Well-Being and Social Development: A National Symposium*, Timber Press, 1992.

Sterling, Arundel, et al., 'Criteria for human exposure to humidity in occupied buildings,' *ASHRAE Transactions*, 1985, Vol. 91, Part I.

Ryushi, T., 'The effect of exposure to negative air ions on the recovery of physiological responses after moderate endurance exercise,' *Int. J. Biometeorology*, 1994, 41: 132-136.

Ryushi, T., 'Physiological effects of exposure to negative air ions on the recovery of fatigue after exercise,' *Japan J. Clinical Ecology*, 1997, 6: 34-40.

Ryushi, T., 'Clinical and physiological effects of negative air ions,' *Japan J. Clinical Ecology*, 2001, 10: 70-77.

Ryushi, T. and H. Sasaki, 'Science of air ions (in Japanese),' *Ningen to Rekishi*, 2002, pp. 720.

Ryushi, T. and H. Sasaki, 'The handbook of science of air ions (in Japanese),' *Ningen to Rekishi*, 2003, pp. 496.

Seo, K.H., et al., 'Bactericidal effects of negative air ions on airborne and surface Salmonella enteritidis from an artificially generated aerosol,' *J. of Food Protection*, 2001, Vol. 64, No. 1: 113-116.

Ulrich, R.S., 'Health benefits of gardens in hospitals,' Plants for People, Intl. Exhibition Floriade 2002 (Netherlands).

Ulrich, R.S., et al., 'Stress recovery during exposure to natural and urban environments,' *J. of Environ. Psychology*, 1991, 11: 201-230.

Wolverton, B.C. and J.D. Wolverton, 'Interior plants: their influence on airborne microbes inside energy-efficient buildings,' *J. of the Mississippi Academy of Sci.* 1996, 41(2): 99-105.

CHAPTER 4: GARDENING

Beverley, D. and B. Phillips, '*Encyclopedia of Gardening*,' 2000, Parragon Publishing, Bath, United Kingdom.

'Botanical Garden,' University of Bonn. Available from http://www.botanik.uni-bonn.de/botgart/0_lang/engl01.htm (17 May 2004); INTERNET.

Bradlow, H.L., et al. 'Effects of dietary indole-3-carbinol on estradiol metabolism and spontaneous mammary tumors in mice.' *Carcinogenesis* 1994; 12:1571-1574.

Challier B., J.M. Perarnau and J.F. Viel, 'Garlic, onion and cereal fiber as protective factors for breast cancer: a French case-control study.' *Eur. J. Epidemiol*, 14(8):737-47, Dec. 1998.

'Chelsea Physic Garden – London.' Available from http://www.chelseaphysic garden.co.uk (17 May 2004): INTERNET.

Chen, I., et al., 'Indole-3-carbinol and diindolylmethane

as aryl hydrocarbon (Ah) receptor agonists and antagonists in T47D human breast cancer cells,' *Fundamentals of Applied Toxicology* 1996; 30:183.

Dorant, E., P.A. Van Den Brandt and R.A. Goldbohm, 'A prospective cohort study on the relationship between onion and leek consumption, garlic supplement use and the risk of colorectal carcinoma in The Netherlands,' *Carcinogenesis*, 17(3):477-84, March 1996.

Dorsch, W., M. Ettl, G. Hein, et al., 'Antiasthmatic effects of onions. Inhibition of platelet-activating factor-induced bronchial obstruction by onion oils,' *Int. Arch. Allergy Appl. Immunol*, 82(3-4):535-6, 1987.

Dreher, M.I., et al., 'The Traditional and Emerging Role of Nuts in Healthful Diets,' *Nutrition Review* 54(8):241-5, August 1996.

Eissenstat, B., et al., 'Impact of Consuming Peanuts and Peanut Products on Energy and Nutrient Intakes of American Adults,' *Peanut Institute Abstract #432.1* (Pennsylvania State University: University Park, PA).

Ensminger, A.H., M.E. Ensminger, J.E. Kondale, J.R.K. Robson, *Foods & Nutrition Encyclopedia*. Pegus Press, Clovis, California.

Fisher, Michele Ph.D., R.D. and Lachance, Paul Ph.D. 'Nutrition and Health Aspects of Almonds,' Rutgers University, April 1999.

Fraser, G.E., et al., 'A Possible Protective Effect of Nut Consumption on Risk of Coronary Heart Disease,' *Archives of Internal Medicine* 152(7): 1416-24, July 1992.

'Gardening and Horticulture,' *The New Encyclopaedia Britannica*, Vol. 19, 2003, pp. 120, 653-688.

Gaynor, M.L. and J. Hickey, *Dr. Gaynor's Cancer Prevention Program*. Kensington Books, New York, 1999.

Gerhauser, C., et al., 'Cancer chemoprevention potential of sulforamate, a novel analogue of sulforaphane that induces Phase 2 drug-metabolizing enzymes,' *Cancer Research* 1997; 57:272-278.

Gormley, James J., *DHA, A Good Fat: Essential for Life*. New York: Kensington Books, 1999.

'Growth Industry: Organic farming is a budding alternative,' Jilian Mincer, The Kansas City Star, 18 March 2003. Available from http://www.ofrf.org/press/Press@20Clippings/KC.Star.031803.2ppdoc.pdf (25 May 2004): INTERNET.

Haenzel, W., et al., 'A case-control study of large bowel cancer in Japan.' *Journal of the National Cancer Institute* 1980; 64:17-22.

Hu, F.B., et al., 'Frequent Nut Consumption and Risk of Coronary Heart Disease in Women: Prospective Cohort Study,' *British Medical Journal* 317(7169): 1341-5, 14 November 1998.

'Japan's Consumers Are Hungry for Organic Food,' Organic Consumer Association, 15 August 2003. Available from http://www.organicconsumers.org/organic/japan_organic.cfm (25 May 2004): INTERNET.

Kuang, Cliff, 'Farming in the sky,' *Popular Science*, September 2008, pg. 41-47.

Michnovicz, J.J. and H.L. Bradlow, 'Induction of estradiol metabolism by dietary indole-e-carbinol in humans.' *Journal of the National Cancer Institute* 1990; 82:947-949.

'Missouri Botanical Garden,' 1997. Available from http:www.gardenweb.com/gotw/mobat.html (17 May 2004): INTERNET.

Morgan, W.A. and B.J. Clayshulte, 'Pecans lower low-density lipoprotein cholesterol in people with normal lipid levels.' *Journal of the American Dietetic Association*, March 2000; 100(3): 312-318.

Osmundson, Theodore H., *Roof Gardens: History, Design and Construction*. Norton, W. W. & Co., Inc., New York, 1999.

'Oxford and Its Collections: A Garden of Wonders,' University of Oxford, Annual Review 2000/2001. Available from http://www.ox.ac.uk/publicrelations/pubs/annualreview/ar01/08.shtml (17 May 2004): INTERNET.

Thacker, Christopher, *England's Historic Gardens*. 1989,

Templar Publishing Ltd., Surrey, United Kingdom.

Tiwari, R.K., Li Guo, H.L. Bradlow, N.T. Telang, and M. P. Osborne, 'Selective responsiveness of human breast cancer cells to indole-3-carbinol, a chemo-preventive agent.' *Journal of the National Cancer Institute* 1994; 86:126-131.

Verhoeven, D.T., et al., 'Epidemiological studies on brassica vegetables and cancer risk.' *Cancer Epidemiological Biomarkets* 1996; 5:733-748.

Wolverton, B.C. 'Higher Plants for Recycling Human Waste into Food, Potable Water and Revitalized Air in a Closed Life Support System,' NASA Research Report No. 192, John C. Stennis Space Center, Mississippi, August 1980.

Wolverton, B.C. and John D. Wolverton, *Growing Clean Water – Nature's Solution to Water Pollution*, Wolverton Environmental Services, Inc., Picayune, Mississippi, 2001.

Yuesheng Zg, T.W. Kensler, Cheon-Gyu Cho, G.H. Posner, P. Talalay, et al., 'Anticarcinogenic activities of sulforaphane and structurally related synthetic NorbomyL isothiocynates.' *Proceedings of the National Academy of Sciences* 1994; 3147-3150.

CHAPTER 5: MEDICINAL PLANTS

Castleman, Michael, The New Healing Herbs. Rodale, Inc., 2001.

Khan, Alam, et al., 'Cinnamon improves glucose and lipid of people with type II diabetes,' *Diabetes Care Journal*, 2003, Vol. 26: 3715-3718.

Lazarous, J., B. Pomeranz and P. Corey, 'Incidence of adverse drug reactions in hospitalized patients,' *J. Amer. Med. Assoc.*, 1998, 279: 1200-1205.

Ling, H. Tiong H. and Nancy T. Ling, *Green Tea and Its Amazing Health Benefits*. Longevity Press, Houston, TX, 2000.

Mabey, Richard, et al., *The New Age Herbalist*. Simon & Schuster, Inc., New York, 1998.

Mindell, Earl, *Earl Mindell's Herb Bible*. Simon & Schuster, Inc., New York, 1992.

Rindels, Sherry, 'All we have is thyme,' *Horticulure*, 4 April 1997, pp. 37-38.

Starfield, B. 'Is the U.S. health really the best in the world?' *J. Amer. Med. Assoc.*, July 26, 2000, 284(4): 483-485.

Taylor, Leslie, *Herbal Secrets of the Rainforest*. Prima Publishing, Rocklin, CA, 1998.

White, L.B. and S. Foster, *The Herbal Drugstore*. Rodale, Inc., 2000.

CHAPTER 6: PLANTS AND THEIR ROLE IN WATER AND WASTE RECYCLING

Moshiri, G.A. (ed.), *Constructed Wetlands for Water Quality Improvement*. Lewis Publishers, Inc., Ann Arbor, MI, 1993.

Reddy, K.R. and W.H. Smith (eds.), *Aquatic Plants for Water Treatment and Resource Recovery*. Magnolia Publishing Co., Orlando, FL, 1987.

Wolverton, B.C., 'Aquatic Plant/Microbial Filters for Treating Septic Tank Effluent,' D.A. Hammer (ed.), *Constructed Wetlands for Wastewater Treatment*, Lewis Publishing, Inc., Chelsea, MI, 1989, pp. 173-178.

Wolverton, B.C., 'Natural Systems for Wastewater Treatment and Water Reuse for Space and Earthly Applications.' Proceedings of American Water Works Association Research Foundation, Water Reuse Symposium IV, Denver, Colorado, 1987, pp. 729-741.

Wolverton, B.C. and R.C. McCaleb, 'Pennywort and Duckweed Marsh System for Upgrading Wastewater Effluent from a Mechanical Package Plant,' K. R. Reddy and W. H. Smith (eds.), *Aquatic Plants for Wastewater Treatment and Resource Recovery*, Magnolia Publishing, Inc., Orlando, Florida, 1987, pp. 289-294.

Wolverton, B.C., R.C. McDonald and W.R. Duffer, 'Micro-organisms and Higher Plants for Wastewater Treatment,' *Journal of Environmental Quality*, 1983, 12(2): 236-242.

Wolverton, B.C., 'Hybrid Wastewater Treatment System Using Anaerobic Micro-organisms and Reed (*Phragmites communis*).' *Economic Botany*, 36(4): 373-380.

Wolverton, B.C., 'Higher Plants for Recycling Human Waste into Food, Potable Water and Revitalized Air in a Closed Life Support System,' NASA/ERL Research Report No. 192, August 1980.

Wolverton, B.C., R.C. McDonald and R.M. Barlow, 'Application of Vascular Aquatic Plants for Pollution Removal, Energy and Food Production,' J. Tourbier and R. W. Pierson, Jr. (eds.), *Biological Control of Water Pollution*, Univ. of Penn. Press, Philadelphia, PA, 1976, pp. 141-149.

Wolverton, B.C. and D.D. Harrison, 'Aquatic Plants for Removal of Mevinphos from the Aquatic Environment,' *Journal of the Mississippi Academy of Science*, 1973, 19: 84-88.

NASA – John C Stennis Space Center, Mississippi, Wastewater Monitoring Data, 1976-1996.

Wolverton, B.C. and John D. Wolverton, *Growing Clean Water: Nature's Solution to Water Pollution*. Wolverton Environmental Services, Inc., Picayune, MS, 2001.

Glossary of Terms

absorption: The passing of chemicals or other substances into plant tissue

adsorption: The adhesion of a gas, liquid or dissolved substance to a surface

aerobic: Requiring oxygen for growth

aerosolized: A gaseous suspension of fine solid or liquid particles

agar: A gelatinous substance derived from seaweeds. An agar plate is a sterile petri dish used to culture microorganisms.

allergen: Substance that induces allergy

allergy: Hypersensitivity; the harmful reaction of antibody to its specific antigen

anaerobic: Growing in the absence of oxygen

angstrom: A unit of length equal to one hundred-millionth (10) of a centimetre; used mainly for specifying the wavelength of radiation, but has been replaced by the nanometre (nm)

aquifer An underground layer of water-bearing permeable rock from which ground water can be extracted using a water well

BTU (British Thermal Unit): A unit of energy equal to the work done by a power of 1000 watts operating for one hour

bioeffluents: Chemicals released during human respiration

bioflavonoids: A group of naturally occurring plant compounds which act primarily as plant pigments and antioxidants

biomass: Refers to living and recently dead biological material that can be used as fuel or for industrial production (wood, crops, etc.)

CFU/plate: Colony forming units of microorganisms grown on agar plates

carbon tetrachloride: A chlorinated organic solvent

diuretic: Anything that promotes the formation of urine by the kidneys

endotoxins: Toxins contained in the cell walls of some microorganisms, especially gram-negative bacteria, that are released when the bacterium dies and are broken down in the body.

expanded clay aggregate: A lightweight highly porous aggregate obtained by heating selected clays at temperatures from 816–1093°C (1500–2000°F). Its porous nature allows for maximum air and water exchange in hydroculture.

flavonoids: A large group of water soluble plant pigments that are beneficial to health

foliage plant: A plant that is grown indoors primarily for the display of its leaves. Although some foliage plants bloom, their flowers are usually insignificant.

free radicals: Atoms or groups of atoms with an odd (unpaired) number of electrons and can be formed when oxygen interacts with certain molecules such as DNA, causing damage

humidity: The amount of water vapour in the air

hydrated aluminosilicates: The chemical structure of zeolite; used in air filtration.

hydroculture: The hydroponic technique of growing houseplants in a water-tight container with support substrate other than soil (for example, expanded clay aggregate), and supplied with a nutrient solution

hydroponics: The technique of growing plants in a medium other than soil whereby water and nutrients flow past plant roots; primarily used in commercial food production

hypersensitivity: Increased sensitivity or allergy to certain substances

inert: Not active

landfill leachate: Liquids that drain from landfills

Jaros Baum & Bolles: Engineering firm serving as mechanical engineers on the construction of the Bank of America building in New York City

mass spectrometer/gas chromatograph: A combination of two analytical chemical instruments used to identify chemicals and determine their concentration levels in air, water, etc.

microbe: A microscopic organism

micron: A unit of length in the metric system equal to one-millionth of a metre; short for micrometre

microorganisms: Microbes; minute forms of life, individually too small to be seen without the aid of a microscope

mutate: To change or undergo mutation

off-gas: To give off or to emit.

photosynthesis: The manufacture of carbohydrate foods (sugars) from carbon dioxide and water in the presence of light and chlorophyll.

phytochemical: A chemical manufactured by a plant.

radioactive carbon tracer: A procedure where carbon molecules in organic chemicals are labeled with radioactive carbon 14 to trace the breakdown path of byproducts.

relative humidity: The amount of water vapour the air is holding expressed as a percentage of the maximum amount the air could potentially hold at that temperature.

rhizosphere: Area around plants influenced by substances excreted by plant roots

spathe: A hood-like bract that partially encloses a spadix (flower spike)

sterols: An important class of organic molecules found in plants, animals and fungii

stomata: Microscopic opening on plant leaves that allow water vapour, oxygen, carbon dioxide and other gases to pass in or out of the leaf

sub-irrigation: The technique of growing plants in soil-filled, water-tight containers in which water is introduced below the surface

symbiotic: A relationship of mutual benefit or dependence

synergistic effect: The effect of two or more chemicals on an organism that is greater than the effect of each chemical individually, or the sum of the individual effects

synthetic: Produced by chemical synthesis rather than of natural origin

tannins: Substances present in seeds and stems of grapes, tea and the bark of some trees

thermal insulation value: The ability of materials to reduce the rate of heat transfer and is measured in R values; the larger their value the less heat loss

thymine: One of the four bases in the nucleic acid of DNA and RNA

thymine dimers: The covalent bonding of two adjacent thymine residues within a DNA molecule, often catalyzed by ultraviolet radiation or chemical mutagenic agents

transpiration: The natural process of water evaporation from plant leaves. Transpiration produces cooling and air movement around plant leaves

ventilation: Dilution of indoor air with outside air

zeolite: Natural volcanic minerals with unique characteristics. Their chemical structure classifies them as hydrated aluminosilicates comprised of hydrogen, oxygen, aluminum and silicon.

Index

R

S

T

U

Photo Credits

Actree Corporation, Matto City, Japan: Pages 46, 47
Albemarle Corporation, Magnolia AR: Page 127
André Trawick, Henderson KY: Pages 73 (below), 75 (right)
Chuck Bargeron, University of Georgia, Bugwood.org: Page 103
City of Chicago IL, Department of Environment: Pages 80, 81
Degussa Corporation, Theodore AL: Page 126
Douglas White, St. Thomas VI: Page 125
Edmunds International, NC: Page 57
First Foliage, Homestead FL: Pages 40, 41
Foliage Design Systems, Orlando FL: Pages 59, 60 (left, right)
Forest and Kim Starr, Makawao HI: Page 107, 113
Green Plants for Green Buildings, Ukiah CA: Page 65 (left)
Gaylord Opryland Resort, Nashville TN: Page 64 (top, below)
J.S. Peterson, USDA-NRCS PLANTS Database: Page 111
Jeff McMillian, USDA-NRCS PLANTS Database: Pages 104, 106
Laila Wessel, Missouri Botanical Garden: Page 73 (top)
Leslie Wallace, Missouri Botanical Garden: Page 75 (left)
Flora of Zimbabwe, Mark Hyde and Bart Wursten: Page 115
National Aeronautics and Space Administration, US (NASA): Pages 28, 29, 30, 32 (top), 34 (top), 123 (top, below), 124
Planterra Corporation, West Bloomfield MI: Pages 38, 39, 42, 51 (top)
Professor Kazuo Yamasaki, Kamakura, Japan: Pages 97, 98 (right), 100, 102, 114
R. A. Howard, USDA-NRCS PLANTS Database: Page 101
Stuart Rose, Poquoson VA: Pages 54, 55, 56
Takenaka Garden Afforestation, Inc.: Pages 62, 63 (left, right)
Umow Lai Pty Ltd, Melbourne, Australia: Page 52
Wolverton Environmental Services, Inc. (WES): Pages 14 (left, right), 15, 34 (below), 45, 49, 50, 61, 65 (right), 74 (all), 76, 77, 78, 87, 99, 105, 108, 109, 112

ILLUSTRATIONS, GRAPHS AND TABLES

Actree Corporation, Matto City, Japan: Page 46 (right)
National Aeronautics and Space Administration, US (NASA): Pages 32 (below), 33, 125
Professor Tové Fjeld, Agricultural University, Oslo, Norway: Page 67
Wolverton Environmental Services, Inc. (WES): Pages 13, 14 (all), 15, 20, 35, 36, 37, 38, 39, 40, 41, 42, 43, 46 (left), 47, 50, 51, 89, 90, 91 (all), 124, 128